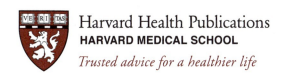

Dear Reader:

Sex. The word can evoke a kaleidoscope of emotions. From love, excitement, and tenderness to longing, anxiety, and disappointment—the reactions are as varied as sexual experiences themselves. What's more, many people will encounter all these emotions and many others in the course of a sex life spanning several decades.

But what is sex, really? On one level, sex is just another hormone-driven bodily function designed to perpetuate the species. Of course, that narrow view underestimates the complexity of the human sexual response. In addition to the biochemical forces at work, your experiences and expectations help shape your sexuality. Your understanding of yourself as a sexual being, your thoughts about what constitutes a satisfying sexual connection, and your relationship with your partner are key factors in your ability to develop and maintain a fulfilling sex life.

The physical transformations your body undergoes as you age also have a major influence on your sexuality. Declining hormone levels and changes in neurological and circulatory functioning may lead to sexual problems such as erectile dysfunction or vaginal pain. Half of men ages 50 and older report at least occasional erection problems. The figure rises to nearly 60% at age 60 and almost 70% at age 70. In addition, many women contend with issues of vaginal dryness and a lagging libido after they pass menopause (when the ovaries stop producing estrogen).

Such physical changes often mean that the intensity of youthful sex may give way to more subdued responses during middle and later life. But the emotional byproducts of maturity—increased confidence, better communication skills, and lessened inhibitions—can help create a richer, more nuanced, and ultimately satisfying sexual experience. However, many people fail to realize the full potential of later-life sex. By understanding the crucial physical and emotional elements that underlie satisfying sex, you can better navigate problems if they arise.

The advice in this report applies broadly to people of all sexual orientations. It will take you through the stages of sexual response and explain how aging affects each. You'll also learn how chronic illnesses, common medications, and emotional issues can influence your sexual capabilities. Finally, you'll find a detailed discussion of various medical treatments, counseling, and self-help techniques to address the most common types of sexual problems.

Sincerely,

Jan Leslie Shifren, M.D.,
*Medical editor*

Suki Hanfling, M.S.W., LICSW
*Medical editor*

# Understanding sexuality

At this stage in your life, you might feel that you know all there is to know about sex. After all, it's probably been many years since you had your first sexual experience. But if you're like a lot of people, you also possess spotty information and faulty beliefs, some of which may be preventing you from fully enjoying your maturing sexuality. To help you build a solid foundation for a fulfilling sex life, here's a quick overview of human sexuality basics.

## How do you define "sex"?

Vaginal intercourse is often given a lofty position as the ultimate sexual event, but clearly the story doesn't end there. Pleasurable activities—from intimacies such as kissing and caressing to more intense types of physical contact designed to produce orgasm—can complement intercourse or stand alone as a means for gratification.

The penis and vagina are not the only tools for sexual enjoyment; people can give and receive intense pleasure without any direct genital-to-genital contact. The mouth, breasts, anal area, hands, and other sensitive spots on the skin are significant sources of erotic sensation. Even the friction of bodies rubbing together, clothed or unclothed, can bring intense sexual pleasure. Sexual activity does not always demand that you have a partner, either. Masturbation, viewing sexually stimulating materials, and creating fantasies all may be avenues for sexual gratification.

## Your sexual anatomy

You know these parts of your body are there, even if you don't know them all by name. The following descriptions and the accompanying diagrams will acquaint you, part by part, with the structures that make up the male and female genitals.

### Female genitals

The appearance of a woman's genital organs is as individual as her face or body type. However, certain basic structures are common to all women (see Figure 1, below). The following parts make up the outer genitals, collectively called the vulva:

■ **Mons pubis:** The fatty mound of tissue that covers the pubic bone. Often called the "mons."

■ **Outer lips (labia majora):** The fleshy folds of skin, fat tissue, and smooth muscle that enclose the vaginal opening. Pubic hair, which may be plentiful or sparse depending on the individual, grows along the outer edges of the labia.

■ **Inner lips (labia minora):** A second set of thinner tissue folds, closer to the vaginal opening. Unlike the pubic hair–studded outer lips, the labia minora have a smooth surface and are rich in tiny blood vessels and nerve endings.

■ **Clitoris:** The most sensitive part of a woman's genital anatomy. This small mound of tissue is located

**Figure 1** Female genitals

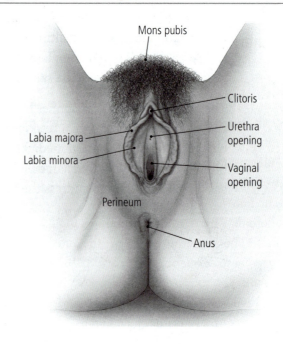

at the point where the upper ends of the labia minora meet, above the vaginal opening. It's constructed from the same tissue as the head of a man's penis (the glans). A soft fold of tissue called the clitoral hood covers the pea-shaped protrusion.

■ **Perineum:** A stretch of hairless, sensitive skin that extends from the bottom of the vaginal opening back to the anus.

Unseen within a woman's body are these structures:

■ **Vagina:** A 3- to 5-inch tube of highly elastic tissue that extends from the vaginal opening to the cervix, at the base of the uterus. Just inside the entrance of the vagina is a ridge of muscles. Normally, the vaginal walls rest against one another. During childbirth, however, the vagina stretches wide enough to allow the baby to pass through. The vagina is lined with a layer of cells that secrete fluid to keep the inner surfaces moist. Blood vessels are plentiful within the vaginal walls, but most of the nerve endings are clustered in the outer third of the vagina.

■ **Cervix:** The knoblike tip of the uterus that forms the opening to the uterus from the vagina. Some women find pressure against the cervix enjoyable during intercourse.

■ **Uterus:** A muscular, fist-sized organ shaped like an upside-down pear. The primary job of the uterus is to harbor a growing fetus during pregnancy. Uterine muscles contract during orgasm, producing a pleasurable sensation.

## Male genitals

Compared with a woman's genitals, a man's sexual anatomy is a straightforward affair (see Figure 2, at right). The primary structure is the penis. This organ does triple duty serving a man's sexual, reproductive, and urinary functions. The penis includes these structures:

■ **Glans:** The head of the penis. The urethral opening at the tip of the glans allows urine and semen to leave the penis.

■ **Corona:** The ridge that separates the glans from the shaft. This and the glans are the most sensitive portions of a man's penis.

■ **Shaft:** The main part of the penis. It houses the corpora cavernosa and the corpus spongiosum.

■ **Corpora cavernosa (erectile bodies):** Two flexible

### Figure 2 Male genitals

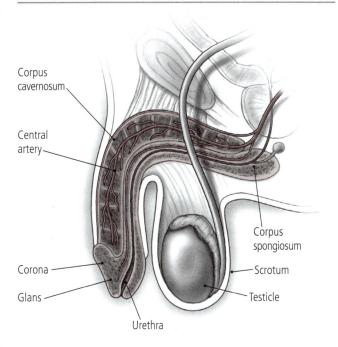

cylinders of erectile tissue that run the length of the penis to support erection.

■ **Corpus spongiosum (spongy body):** A cylindrical body of erectile tissue that surrounds the urethra and includes the glans.

■ **Central artery:** The vessel that supplies blood to erectile tissue in the corpora cavernosa.

■ **Urethra:** A narrow tube that extends the length of the penis and carries both urine and semen out of the body.

In addition to the penis are the following structures:

■ **Scrotum:** The sac of skin at the base of the penis that holds the testes. The scrotum is covered, to varying degrees depending on the individual, with pubic hair.

■ **Testes or testicles:** The reproductive glands that produce sperm.

■ **Prostate gland:** A walnut-sized gland located at the base of the bladder. The prostate produces a milky fluid that carries the sperm out of the body during ejaculation.

# The phases of sexual response

In the heat of sexual excitement, few people want to bother deciphering the dynamics of their sexual response. However, in cooler moments, acquainting yourself with the physiology of sex can offer clues to help you heighten your pleasure and improve your sexual capabilities.

The process that begins with the first glimmer of desire and culminates in the series of pleasurable rhythmic contractions we know as orgasm can be divided into four distinct phases. Each is characterized by a set of anatomic and physiologic changes. The four phases are as follows:

■ **Desire.** Also called lust or libido, desire is the wish for sex. A sight, sound, taste, touch, or smell may spark it. Or it may be ignited by a memory or fantasy. Desire may occur before any physical signs of sexual readiness take place in your body or in response to sexual stimulation. Desire often leads to arousal and orgasm, but this isn't always the case. Arousal can also lead to desire, and desire can linger on its own indefinitely.

■ **Arousal.** During arousal, blood floods into the genitals, triggering the man's penis to stiffen and the woman's labia, clitoris, and upper vagina to swell. Moisture begins seeping from the vaginal lining, creating lubrication. The vagina lengthens, the uterus rises, and the inner and outer lips pull apart, exposing the vaginal opening. The man's testicles pull closer to his body, and his scrotum becomes thicker. In both sexes, breathing and heart rate accelerate, muscles throughout the body tense, the skin flushes, and nipples become erect.

■ **Orgasm.** When muscle tension and genital engorgement peak, a series of rhythmic contractions occurs in the sex organs. The contractions force the congested blood out of the tissues and back into circulation. Along with this comes an abrupt release of muscle tension and a pleasurable sensation. In a man, penile contractions expel semen out of the urethra; this is known as ejaculation. Some women also release fluid during orgasm. Although this fluid comes out of the urethra, it's not urine. Glands located in the same area as the G-spot (see "The G-spot," at left) may produce the fluid.

■ **Resolution.** Following orgasm, heart rate and blood pressure gradually return to their normal levels. In a man, the penis becomes flaccid; in a woman, sex organs gradually return to their unaroused state. After orgasm, it takes some time before an individual can have another orgasm. For a woman, this stage may pass quickly, allowing her to have multiple orgasms in a short span of time if stimulation continues. A man generally needs to wait longer—from several minutes to hours or days, depending on his age—before he is able to ejaculate again.

While it's possible to identify these discrete parts of the sexual response cycle, not every sexual encounter needs to progress through all four phases in an orderly manner, or necessarily include orgasm. This is true for both women and men.

## Differences in male and female response

In the decades after William H. Masters and Virginia E. Johnson introduced the concept of the stages of sexual response in 1966, it was widely assumed that a woman's response closely mimicked that of a man. More

### The G-spot

The G-spot, or Grafenberg spot, named after the gynecologist who first identified it, is a mound of super-sensitive spongelike tissue located within the roof of the vagina, just inside the entrance. Proper stimulation of the G-spot can produce intense orgasms. Because of its difficult-to-reach location and the fact that it is most successfully stimulated manually, the G-spot is not routinely activated for most women during vaginal intercourse. While this has led some skeptics to doubt its existence, research has demonstrated that a different sort of tissue does exist in this location.

You must be sexually aroused to be able to locate your G-spot. To find it, try rubbing your finger in a beckoning motion along the roof of your vagina while you're in a squatting or sitting position, or have your partner massage the upper surface of your vagina until you notice a particularly sensitive area. Some women tend to be more sensitive and can find the spot easily, but for others it's difficult. If you can't easily locate it, you shouldn't worry.

During intercourse, many women feel that the G-spot can be most easily stimulated when the man enters from behind. For couples dealing with erection problems, play involving the G-spot can be a positive addition to lovemaking. Oral stimulation of the clitoris combined with manual stimulation of the G-spot can give a woman a highly intense orgasm.

**Table 1** Possible age-related sexual changes in women and men

| | WOMEN | MEN |
|---|---|---|
| **Physical changes** | Decreased blood flow to the genitals. Lower levels of estrogen and testosterone. Thinning of the vaginal lining. Loss of vaginal elasticity and muscle tone. | Decreased testosterone. Reduced blood flow to the penis. Less sensitivity in the penis. |
| **Desire** | Decreased libido. Fewer sexual thoughts and fantasies. | Decreased libido. Fewer sexual thoughts and fantasies. |
| **Arousal** | Slower arousal. Reduced vaginal lubrication and less expansion of the vagina during arousal. Less blood congestion in the clitoris and lower vagina. Diminished clitoral sensitivity. | Greater difficulty achieving an erection, maintaining an erection, or both. Erections aren't as rigid. |
| **Orgasm** | Delayed or absent orgasm. Less intense orgasms. Fewer and sometimes painful uterine contractions. | Longer time required to reach orgasm. Smaller volume of semen and less forceful ejaculation. Less intense orgasms. |
| **Resolution** | Body returns more rapidly to an unaroused state. | Body returns more rapidly to an unaroused state. More time is needed between erections. |

recently, however, researchers have focused attention on women's sexual response. Researchers at the University of British Columbia have found that the patterns of response may vary widely between the sexes.

For example, when it comes to desire, male and female sexual responses diverge. The sex drive of men tends to be goal-oriented, setting its sights on intercourse and orgasm. This drive is propelled by frequent sexual fantasies and thoughts. Although women are equally capable of strong sexual urges, typically desire manifests itself as a more diffuse, sometimes elusive, drive. As they age, women are more likely to become aroused by demonstrations of emotional intimacy—such as acts that reveal caring, commitment, or tenderness—rather than sexual fantasies alone.

This school of thought also contends that women may experience the stages of sexual response in a nonlinear manner. That is, arousal may need to occur before desire appears. In turn, the emotional intimacy that typically occurs between partners following lovemaking ("afterplay") can trigger a woman's desire for sex in the future. Women may also find that arousal and orgasm progress in the form of a series of rolling hills, rather than as a steady buildup to a dramatic peak followed by a steep drop. But men can also experience flagging desire and arousal, particularly if they have had surgery or other treatments for prostate cancer. They too may find that activities that cause arousal (including taking medications for erectile dysfunction) can in turn stimulate desire.

# The impact of aging

Advancing years leave their mark on the body, mind, and emotions. Some of these changes are for the better, while others are less desirable. Sex is no exception. Many of the physical changes that come with age have noticeable effects on the sex organs and the sexual cycle (see Table 1, above). Thus, the careful lovemaking of a 70-something couple may bear little resemblance to the lusty pairings of 20-year-olds. This isn't necessarily a bad thing. Greater experience, fewer inhibitions, and a deeper understanding of your needs and those of your partner can more than compensate for the consequences of aging, such as slower arousal, softer erections, reduced vaginal lubrication, and less intense orgasms. And these physical changes can provide an impetus for developing a new and satisfying style of lovemaking—one that's based more on extended foreplay and less on intercourse and orgasm.

### The role of menopause

While midlife brings many changes for women, menopause is clearly a physical milestone. Menopause and the preceding months or years (known as perimenopause) are marked by hormonal fluctuations, which can provoke a host of symptoms, such as hot flashes, vaginal dryness, and changes in body shape (see Table 2, page 6). Many of these effects—vaginal changes and loss of libido, in particular—can wreak havoc on a woman's sex life.

### Table 2 The rise and fall of women's sex hormones

| | ESTROGEN | PROGESTERONE | TESTOSTERONE |
|---|---|---|---|
| What is the function of this hormone? | The "female" hormone, estrogen causes the uterine lining to thicken during the menstrual cycle. It stimulates the growth of breast tissue and maintains blood flow to and lubrication of the vagina. It has many other effects, including maintaining bone density and keeping the skin and vaginal lining elastic. | Progesterone prepares the lining of the uterus for implantation of a fertilized egg and helps maintain early pregnancy. If pregnancy does not occur, the loss of progesterone causes the uterine lining to shed. | Commonly known as the "male" hormone, testosterone is also important to women's sexual health. It plays a key role in the production of estrogen in women, contributes to libido, and may help maintain bone density and muscle mass. |
| How do perimenopause and menopause affect this hormone? | During perimenopause, levels fluctuate and become unpredictable. Eventually, production stops completely. | Progesterone production ceases when ovulation stops. | Testosterone production peaks in a woman's 20s, then declines gradually. By menopause, the level is at half of its peak. The ovaries continue to make testosterone even after estrogen production stops. Testosterone production from the adrenal glands also declines with aging, but continues after menopause. |
| What symptoms may occur as a result? | **Estrogen overproduction:** bloating, breast tenderness.<br>**Estrogen withdrawal:** hot flashes, night sweats, palpitations, headaches, insomnia, fatigue, bone loss, vaginal dryness. | **Lack of progesterone:** periods may become irregular, longer, or heavier during perimenopause. | **Testosterone decline:** unknown. |

Even so, women don't have to be at the mercy of their hormones. Lifestyle changes, vaginal lubricants and moisturizers, or hormone therapy (see Table 8, page 33) may help alleviate many of these problems.

### Is there a male menopause?

The answer is both yes and no. In the strictest sense, men don't normally experience the precipitous drop in reproductive hormones that marks a woman's midlife. Although testosterone—the hormone responsible for a man's libido and fertility as well as his deep voice and facial hair—does taper off as a man ages, the process happens gradually. After about age 25, the level of testosterone in the blood diminishes by an average of 1% each year. But this fact means little in itself because actual levels can fluctuate dramatically from person to person. It's not impossible for a man in his 70s to be able to father a child.

That said, men may notice changes in their sex lives after they reach their 50s. Erections may require more direct stimulation, the need to ejaculate is less urgent, and the rest period between ejaculations grows longer. However, none of these effects need interfere with a satisfying sex life, provided the man and his partner understand these changes and integrate them into their lovemaking. A couple may find that less penile sensitivity means that the man may be able to enjoy a wider range of erotic sensations and maintain his erection longer. And his experience may pay off in improved sexual technique and a better understanding of what will please his partner.

### Testing testosterone

Many men have no doubt seen ad campaigns urging them to ask their doctor about testosterone testing and treatment if they feel tired, have trouble concentrating, and notice a drop in sex drive.

According to guidelines released in 2010 by the Endocrine Society, "red flags" that raise the possibility of low testosterone include a low libido, erectile dysfunction, a low sperm count, loss of body hair, and hot flashes. Other signs that could prompt your clinician to suspect low testosterone are poor concentration and memory; feeling sad or blue; insomnia; decreased energy, motivation, initiative, or self-confidence; decreased muscle mass and increased fat; and diminished physical or work performance. However, these symptoms are also common in men with normal testosterone levels.

But determining if a man is truly deficient in testosterone is far from simple. For one thing, total testosterone fluctuates quite a bit during the day. Testosterone levels are highest in the morning, although this effect is less pronounced in older men. To get the best result, physicians generally draw blood for testosterone lab tests between 7 a.m. and 10 a.m. And while normal testosterone ranges from about 270 to 1070 nanograms per deciliter (ng/dL), a reading under 270 doesn't necessarily mean a man is deficient. The definition of "low" depends on the local standard adopted by the health care provider and the testing lab. The line at which you cross into "low T" can be 230, 250, 270, or 300. Also, the measured testosterone levels vary from test to test and from lab to lab.

The main issue with the total testosterone lab test is that a lot of the hormone it measures is not biologically active in the body. A small percentage of the total testosterone, from 1% to 2%, floats around on its own in the blood. This "free" testosterone is biologically active. About half the remaining hormone is loosely attached to a protein called albumin. This kind of testosterone, like free testosterone, is potentially available for work. The two, together, represent the "bioavailable" hormone the body's tissues actually respond to.

But anywhere from 40% to 70% of total testosterone travels around with a protein called SHBG. It is bound so tightly to SHBG that it can't be released, and therefore isn't available to your cells.

As a result, a large portion of your measured total testosterone actually may be biologically inactive. This can be misleading in certain circumstances. Experts say that if your levels are borderline low, you don't know if it's real or if it's a variation in SHBG levels. For example, if a man's SHBG is on the high side, his total testosterone may be solidly in the normal range even though his biologically active testosterone is low. The opposite is true, too: if the SHBG is low, a man's total testosterone level may look abnormally low even though his bioavailable testosterone level is well within the norm.

Why not just test free testosterone and avoid the whole SHBG issue? Unfortunately, lab tests for free testosterone are also unreliable—even more so than tests for total testosterone. In fact, a study by the Endocrine Society found that measurements of free testosterone in the same blood sample can vary by a factor of five.

To obtain a clear-cut diagnosis—either confirming low T or ruling it out—work with a physician who understands the complexities of testosterone testing and can interpret the results in light of a man's symptoms. A careful evaluation could involve testosterone measurements on more than one day, as well as tests for levels of hormones related to testosterone. And don't be afraid to ask for a second opinion.

Even when lab tests don't show clear testosterone deficiency, the final decision to offer treatment is a judgment call. If a man has symptoms of testosterone deficiency and a low-normal testosterone level, some providers will consider prescribing of a trial of testosterone replacement. The drug is most widely available as a patch worn on the arm or torso, a gel rubbed into the upper arms or thighs, or a tablet placed inside the upper gums.

But be sure to discuss the potential risks and benefits with your health care provider. Some men who take testosterone develop acne, swelling or tenderness of the breasts, or swelling in the ankles. Your clinician should monitor your red blood cell counts, as an increase in these cells can raise your risk of developing a blood clot.

Some physicians remain wary of prescribing testosterone supplements to men with active prostate cancer, those who have had it in the past, or those who may be at higher risk for it in the future. The reason: In men with advanced prostate cancer, blocking testosterone slows down tumor growth. The concern is whether boosting hormone levels could activate early cancer or speed up tumor growth in men who already have prostate cancer. Others maintain that the risk remains unproven. If you do try testosterone supplementation, remember it's just a trial run. If you don't notice any improvement in your symptoms within three to six months, you might as well stop the treatment.

## What is sexual dysfunction?

Sexual dysfunction can be defined as any aspect of your sexual response that causes you significant dissatisfaction or distress. The focus here is not on the problem itself, but on the fact that the condition is troubling to the people involved. For example, if both members of a couple are content to live without sexual activity, then such conditions as erectile dysfunction or vaginal dryness would not be considered sexual dysfunction. Likewise, a woman who is not involved in a relationship may not be concerned by her low libido. On the other hand, if she finds a partner who has a more active sex drive, her lack of interest will probably become a problem.

Experts usually divide types of sexual dysfunction into male and female issues. Under these headings, they define more specific problems based loosely on three of the four phases of sexual response: desire, arousal, and orgasm. Despite these distinctions, sexual problems are often complex and incorporate elements from more than one category.

Types of sexual dysfunction that occur in women include the following:

- **Sexual desire disorder.** An absence of sexual fantasies, thoughts, or behavior that results in personal distress. Sexual aversion disorder, which is the avoidance of certain types of sexual activity because of severe anxiety, almost to the point of phobia, falls under this heading as well, although it usually has its roots in different psychological issues.
- **Sexual arousal disorder.** A lack of sexual excitement or awareness of sexual pleasure, including absence of vaginal lubrication and other physical indications of arousal, that leads to distress.
- **Orgasmic disorder.** Difficulty or delay in reaching orgasm, or absence of orgasm after sufficient stimulation that causes distress.
- **Sexual pain disorders.** Genital pain during sexual intercourse (dyspareunia). This category includes nonspecific pain in the vulva (vulvodynia) and involuntary tightening of the vagina (vaginismus) that prevents penetration.

Types of sexual dysfunction that occur in men include the following:

- **Sexual desire disorder.** An absence of sexual fantasies, thoughts, or behavior that causes personal distress. Although this problem is more common in women than in men, about one in seven men reported low libido in a survey published in *The Journal of the American Medical Association*, and the proportion rises with age.
- **Erectile dysfunction.** The inability to produce an erection that's sufficient for intercourse. Although this is a relatively uncommon problem for young men, about 44% of men ages 40 to 70 have partial or complete erectile dysfunction (see page 22).
- **Ejaculatory disorders.** These include several orgasmic disorders. Rapid or premature ejaculation occurs when the man ejaculates before penetration, immediately or soon after penetration, or before the couple has achieved a mutually satisfying sexual experience. Delayed ejaculation, when a man has a normal erection but isn't able to reach orgasm, is less common, but tends to increase with age. Certain antidepressant medications, particularly selective serotonin reuptake inhibitors (SSRIs), can cause delayed ejaculation.

# Trends in sexual behavior among older adults

The oldest members of the baby boom generation were in their 20s during the heyday of the 1960s sexual revolution, which was fostered in part by the advent of the birth control pill. During that time, sexual attitudes and practices shifted dramatically. Now these boomers are once again transforming the sexual landscape, challenging views on sexuality and aging. Contrary to what some people believe, many people in their 60s and beyond are sexually active.

In 2007, *The New England Journal of Medicine* published a study about sexual behavior and activity in older adults. The authors surveyed a national sample of 3,005 adults ages 57 to 85, which they then analyzed by three age groups: ages 57 to 64; ages 65 to 74, and ages 75 to 85. Below is a summary of their findings.

## How often and how important?

Nearly three-quarters of those in the youngest group were sexually active, as were just over half of those in the middle group. Among people in the oldest group, sexual activity (defined as having sex with a partner within the past year) dropped to 26%. But even in that oldest group, just over half of those who were sexually active reported that they had sex at least two to three times per month, and nearly a quarter said they had sex once a week or more.

Over all, 35% of women rated sex as "not at all important," compared with 13% of men. Sex became less important with age: 41% of those in the oldest age group rated it as not important, compared with 25% of those in the middle group and 15% of those in the youngest group.

## Contributing factors

Not surprisingly, one of the major factors associated with the likelihood of being sexually active was the availability of a partner. At any given age, women were less likely than men to be married or to be involved in an intimate relationship—a difference that rose sharply with age. In the oldest group, 78% of the men had a spouse or other intimate partner, compared with 40% of the women. This difference likely stems from the facts that men are, on average, married to younger women and that men die at younger ages than women (see "Lack of a partner," page 11).

People who rated themselves as having poor health were less sexually active, and over all, physical health was more closely linked to many sexual problems than was age alone. In particular, diabetes stood out as interfering with sexual function for both genders. People with health problems who were sexually active were more likely to report sexual prob-

### Table 3 Most common sexual problems in middle-aged and older men

| PROBLEM | % WITH THE PROBLEM (% BOTHERED BY IT) |
|---|---|
| Difficulty achieving or maintaining and erection | 37 (90) |
| Lack of interest in sex | 28 (65) |
| Climaxing too quickly | 28 (71) |
| Anxiety about performance | 27 (75) |
| Inability to climax | 20 (73) |

### Table 4 Most common sexual problems in middle-aged and older women

| PROBLEM | % WITH THE PROBLEM (% BOTHERED BY IT) |
|---|---|
| Lack of interest in sex | 43 (61) |
| Difficulty with lubrication | 39 (68) |
| Inability to climax | 34 (59) |
| Finding sex not pleasurable | 23 (64) |
| Pain (most commonly felt at the vaginal opening during entry) | 17 (97) |

lems. Tables 3 and 4 (see page 9) summarize the most common sexual problems reported by the men and women who responded to the survey, as well as the percentage of those with the problem who were troubled by it. According to the authors, older adults who have medical problems or who are considering treatment that might affect their sex lives should be counseled based on their health rather than their age.

Here are a few other findings from the study:

- Among people who had a spouse or other intimate partner who had not had sex for three months or longer, the most common reason cited for the lack of sex was a male partner's physical health.
- 14% of men and 1% of women said they'd taken prescription or nonprescription medication or supplements to boost their sexual function in the past year.
- 38% of men and 22% of women reported discussing sex with a physician since they turned 50.

Two other studies offer more detail about the prevalence of these common complaints. The Massachusetts Male Aging Study, which involved more than 1,700 men ages 40 to 70 living near Boston, found that over all, about 43% of the men had some degree of erectile dysfunction. While just 1% of men in their 40s have this problem, nearly half of men ages 75 and older have complete erectile dysfunction, meaning they are never able to achieve an erection sufficient for intercourse (see Figure 3, at right).

A nationwide survey of more than 31,000 women ages 18 and older confirmed earlier findings that about 43% of women have some type of sexual problem. But only 12% said they felt distressed about the problem, as described in the study, which was published in the journal *Obstetrics and Gynecology* in 2008. Distressing sexual problems peak in midlife, with middle-aged women reporting more distress than younger or older women. Researchers found that one in eight women ages 45 to 64 felt distressed about her lack of sexual desire, and about one in 15 was concerned about arousal and orgasm problems.

**Figure 3** Aging and erectile dysfunction

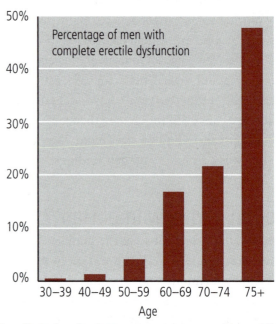

Erectile dysfunction becomes more common with age. While roughly 1% of men ages 40 to 49 have complete erectile dysfunction, nearly 17% of those in their 60s have this condition.
*Source:* Archives of Internal Medicine, *Jan. 23, 2006 pp. 207–12.*

# Emotional and social issues

"The brain is the body's most important sex organ." This oft-repeated statement bears more than a little truth. While the initial prerequisites for sexual activity are physiological—functional sex organs, adequate hormone levels, and the ability to respond to erotic cues—these elements don't guarantee sexual satisfaction. A number of other factors can make you more vulnerable to sexual problems.

## Lack of a partner

For older people, not having a partner is common. By age 65, many people find themselves alone, typically through either divorce or widowhood.

The partner gap is a particular problem for American women because their average life span (81 years) is about five years longer than that of men. Because American women marry men who are on average three years older, that can mean even more time alone. Should a woman want to remarry, her chance of finding a new mate in her age bracket dwindles yearly; there are, on average, only seven men for every 10 women ages 65 and above.

Finally, starting a new sexual relationship after the loss of a partner can present its own dilemmas. People often fear that they will not become aroused or be able to have an orgasm with a different partner. They also may be self-conscious about baring their body in front of someone new. Because a new relationship may come along months or years after their last sexual relationship, some individuals feel anxious that they have "forgotten how to have sex" or that "the equipment doesn't work anymore." For those who have lost a much-loved spouse, feelings of guilt or disloyalty at starting a new relationship can be overwhelming.

## Relationship issues

Tension and emotional distance in a relationship can be detrimental to a couple's sex life. In many cases, serious conflict or lack of emotional intimacy is at the root of a sexual problem. Other times, a sexual issue strains a couple's ability to get along. The following issues are often connected to sexual problems.

■ **Anger and frustration.** Accumulated anger, hurt, disappointment, and resentment can fester, destroying closeness between partners. These pent-up feelings almost always diminish desire. For both men and women, anger and frustration can interfere with arousal. Likewise, the breakdown of trust can be devastating to a person's ability to enjoy sex. In addition, one member of the couple may subconsciously withhold sex as a way of expressing anger or to maintain the upper hand in a situation where he or she feels otherwise powerless.

■ **Poor communication.** Communication is essential for partners to build the trust needed for a successful sexual relationship. By talking frankly about your feelings and wishes, you and your partner can collaborate on finding solutions to issues and can prevent resentments from piling up. When conversation breaks down, anger and resentment are likely to build.

Dialogue is especially vital as physical changes take place. Vaginal dryness or erection difficulties can be wrongly perceived as lack of attraction to the partner or waning interest in sex, which can trigger feelings of rejection and resentment. By articulating feelings, couples can sort out the physiological factors from the emotional and relationship issues, and address each appropriately (see "Talking to your partner," page 45).

■ **Boredom.** Once the honeymoon period is over, almost every couple has to contend with some sexual boredom. The person who was once so electrifyingly mysterious and exciting to you may become as comfortable—and as alluring—as an old shoe. Sex may not even seem worth the trouble when you're facing the same old lovemaking routines.

When sexual activity wanes, other types of physical affection often fade, too. This lack of any kind of physical connection or affection often contributes to emotional distance between you and your partner. As a result, it's all the more difficult to resume sexual intimacy later on. But because inhibitions often lessen with age, sex at 50 or 60 can include a level of creativity, passion, and playfulness you wouldn't have dreamed of in your younger years.

■ **Infidelity.** People have affairs for many reasons, including dissatisfaction, a quest for newness, or a need for self-affirmation. This yearning may arise from a need to banish midlife drudgery, a desire to find out what sex is like with someone else, or an urge to recapture the heart-pounding sexual highs of youth. Other times, an individual seeks out a new partner to meet unfulfilled emotional needs. Sometimes sexual dysfunction in the marriage contributes to affairs. For example, men who have erection difficulties or women who can't reach orgasm may seek out new lovers to prove that the sexual problem is their spouse's doing, not their own. Likewise, the partners of those with sexual difficulties may try to seek reassurance that they're still sexually appealing in the arms of someone else.

The reverberations of an affair can extend throughout a couple's relationship like ripples on a pond. Sometimes the straying partner isn't able to respond sexually to his or her spouse because of guilt over the affair, fatigue from juggling two sexual relationships, or a negative comparison of the spouse with the new lover. If the spouse discovers the affair, he or she is likely to withdraw both emotionally and physically.

An affair can be a serious, sometimes fatal, blow to a relationship. However, it's possible for a couple not only to survive infidelity, but also to grow from this painful experience. To do this, though, both partners must face the personal and relationship issues that may have contributed to the infidelity. Couples therapy is a good place to turn for help in doing this. Sex therapy can also be useful if the affair has either caused, or resulted in part from, sexual problems.

## Performance anxiety

Defined as an overwhelming concern about sexual performance that obscures pleasure and leads to sexual dysfunction, performance anxiety is a particularly insidious issue affecting aging couples. Performance anxiety becomes a problem for both men and women as they move into their 50s.

In men, it's the most common psychological contributor to erectile dysfunction. Here's how the problem often develops. The natural effects of aging dictate that a man needs more time and direct penile stimulation for an erection. Medications and cardiovascular disease may also contribute to erection difficulties. If a man continues to expect the instantaneous rock-hard erections of his 20s, he may equate this change in his physical response with the end of his virility. Once he makes this erroneous leap in his thinking, the problem often snowballs. After a few incidences of erection failure, embarrassment and feelings of defeat leave him unwilling to try again. He may withdraw from all forms of physical intimacy to avoid failure or his fear of not performing. In turn, his partner feels rejected and fears that she or he is no longer attractive enough to sexually excite him. She or he may also suspect him of having an affair.

If this happens, the partner may shy away from touching his penis directly, out of fear that he will feel pressured to perform. Paradoxically, any reticence denies the man just the type of direct stimulation that he needs to achieve an erection. The result is that an addressable physical issue becomes a morass of anger, resentment, and frustration.

Women experience performance anxiety in different ways. Performance anxiety is common in women who have experienced pain during sex (dyspareunia) in the past. They may be worried that sex will be

### Mental health affects sexuality, too

A negative self-image isn't always rooted in your appearance. Career setbacks or other disappointments can lead to feelings of failure and depression, both of which sap desire. For men, episodes of impotence can undercut confidence in their masculinity. No matter what its cause, a poor self-image can take a toll on your sex life. When performance anxiety develops as a result, it can spark a downward spiral of repeated sexual failure and diminishing self-esteem. Correcting this problem demands serious attention to its origin.

uncomfortable again, and this anxiety can decrease lubrication or cause involuntary tightening of the vaginal muscles. In turn, this makes sex more painful, which heightens anxiety and further interferes with lubrication. Women also worry about how long it might take to reach orgasm, which may interfere with experiencing maximum pleasure during sex and make orgasm more difficult. Ultimately, some women decide to avoid sex entirely.

The frank discussion of sexuality that has become commonplace in women's magazines and on daytime television can also contribute to performance anxiety. This openness has had the unintended consequence of making some women worry that they do not respond quickly or intensely enough to be considered a "good lover."

## Body image and self-esteem

Gravity is not kind to your body as you age. Nor is childbirth, a fatty diet, lack of exercise, or the hormone declines that lead to muscle loss, loose skin, and thinning hair. Worry about having your partner see your sagging skin or generous waistline can discourage you from having sex, or you may demand that sex take place only under the covers, with the lights out. Needless to say, these conditions don't leave much room for a sense of closeness or inspired lovemaking. Often, a preoccupation with your appearance while making love will prevent you from initiating or responding to sexual advances.

Relationship conflicts can ensue. When one partner needs constant reassurance about his or her attractiveness and becomes overly sensitive to perceived criticism, it can foster mutual resentment.

By shifting your focus away from your perceived flaws to your attributes, you can boost your self-esteem and establish your own standards for attractiveness. Think back on what it was that made you attractive in your younger years. Was it your soulful brown eyes, your crooked smile, or maybe your infectious laugh? Chances are, those qualities are still as appealing as ever.

Also, try directing your attention to the experience of giving and receiving pleasure during sex. This can help you find the confidence to give yourself over to the experience. Great sex is often the outgrowth of a deep emotional connection—something that's not guaranteed by having a perfect body.

For people who are overweight, exercise can help foster weight loss, as well as provide a mental and physical boost. Even if you lose only a small amount of weight, being active can tone your body, which can improve your body image and, in turn, your sexual interest and response.

## Expectations and past experiences

Your sexuality is a natural drive that's with you from birth, but your family, your culture, your religious background, the media, and your peers shape your attitudes toward sex. As you become an adult, your own experiences further influence your sexuality. The result for many is a healthy enjoyment of sex, but others may have more mixed feelings.

For example, women—particularly those who came of age before the so-called sexual revolution in the '60s—may cling to the notion that it is improper for "nice girls" to initiate and enjoy sex too enthusiastically. This belief can be damaging for both partners. The woman may feel uncomfortable seeking pleasure, and her partner may interpret this lack of enthusiasm as a reflection of her feelings about him or her.

Inexperience and embarrassment over discussing sexual matters may hamper people from fully expressing themselves sexually. For example, intercourse alone without direct clitoral stimulation does not give many women the kind of stimulation they need for fulfilling sex, and uneasiness about discussing the problem prevents some couples from developing techniques that could offer greater pleasure. Compounding the problem, childhood taboos against masturbation may prevent a woman from discovering this means to her sexual pleasure, leaving her unable to direct her partner in this regard. A woman may find it easier to forgo her own pleasure than to confront these matters.

Alternately, a man may feel his self-worth depends on his ability to please his partner. His focus during sex, therefore, is on performing rather than experiencing his own pleasure. If his partner doesn't immediately respond to his efforts, feelings of inadequacy can pervade the relationship, eroding the couple's bond and leading to performance anxiety.

During the early years of a couple's relationship, such missed connections are often masked by priorities outside the bedroom, such as building a marriage, raising a family, and launching a career. However, midlife may be a turning point. Upon reaching menopause, the long-unsatisfied woman might greet the physical changes in her body as a sign that her sexual "duties" are fulfilled. If her partner is still interested in sex, a conflict is likely to erupt.

A much more hopeful scenario is also possible. Midlife and later may be a time when a woman's sexuality blossoms. Women often gain confidence as they mature, and they may be more willing to ask for what they want sexually. Menopause means that women no longer have to worry about pregnancy (or birth control). Often, children are grown and family responsibilities have eased, allowing a couple to engage in more relaxed and spontaneous lovemaking. In addition, the changes a man is experiencing during these years, such as slower erections and longer time before ejaculation, lend themselves to the kind of pleasurable play that a couple may have been missing out on before. For a couple wishing to embark on the more positive course, the key is to begin to unravel negative patterns. To do this, you must open up a dialogue.

## Stress and lifestyle issues

Stress and fatigue are major libido sappers. During midlife, stress can hit from any direction. Challenging teenagers, financial worries, aging parents, concern about your health or that of a loved one, and career woes are common. With so many demands on your time and attention, you and your partner may neglect to nurture your relationship, which can cause your sexual connection to fray.

Sheer lack of time—and failure to prioritize your relationship—is often a major factor. After all, if you were working on a hobby you loved, you probably wouldn't wait until the very end of the day to make time for it. The physical changes in sexual response that occur in both men and women as they age mean that it will take you and your partner more time to become aroused and reach orgasm than it did in your younger years. You may find it hard to squeeze an extended lovemaking session into an already packed day. If a couple typically waits until bedtime to have sex, exhaustion also can become an obstacle.

Stress has a particularly deleterious effect on libido. Whereas some people can sometimes use sex to relax, others more often need to be relaxed in order to enjoy sex. This mismatch can create conflict for a couple.

Sexual issues brought on solely by stress and fatigue often can be remedied simply by taking a short vacation or even a weekend away. If you and your partner are able to resume pleasurable lovemaking in a pressure-free environment, it's quite possible that the underpinnings of your sexual relationship are sound.

Midlife and after is also a time when profound lifestyle changes take place. Events such as retirement and children leaving home can upset decades-long patterns in a couple's life. Many couples go through a period of adjustment when they retire. For example, if one person is used to being in the house alone much of the time, his or her feeling of control over the domain can be threatened by the partner's constant presence.

One bonus is that retirement or changes in working habits may allow you and your partner the opportunity to do more pleasurable things together and engage in leisurely and more spontaneous lovemaking. One danger, however, is that couples who begin spending a lot of time together may stop making an effort to include novelty as well as romance in their relationship.

Chronic illness is a major cause of sexual difficulties. People who are ill may find that a condition or its treatment causes sexual difficulties, while healthy partners may worry that sexual activity will make their loved one's condition worse. The fatigue and stress of the caretaker role may also dampen desire. In addition, sexual interest may wane for both partners if their caretaker-patient relationship begins to feel too much like that of a parent and child. Pain, exhaustion and worry about illness can either interfere with or totally inhibit sexual desire. During this time of life, many people also experience the loss of someone close. Grieving may make it difficult to enjoy anything pleasurable, including sex. ♥

# Health problems and sexuality

Long-term medical conditions compound the sexual issues that men and women already face during the natural aging process. Heart disease, diabetes, cancer, and arthritis are just some of the illnesses that can have a serious, lasting impact on your sexuality. Treatments can also alter sexual functioning. What's more, the emotional effects of an illness often weigh as heavily as the physical ones. One or both members of the couple may experience depression, which is a major contributor to sexual problems.

Among people surveyed for the aging and sexuality study described earlier, people who rated their health as fair or poor were also more likely to report sexual problems, including difficulty with arousal or lubrication, pain, and lack of pleasure.

When you're first confronted with an illness, things may look bleak. But many people are able to resume a satisfying sex life after an adjustment phase. The first step to overcoming these challenges is to investigate the potential effects of the disease and treatment on your sex life. This section provides an overview of some common conditions and how they affect sexuality in later life. But it is also important to discuss these issues with a health care provider—and your partner.

Keep in mind, too, that there are many ways to maintain physical intimacy. Some couples find that they can have a satisfying relationship without intercourse. However, even in the absence of sexual contact, preserving other forms of affection—such as hand-holding and cuddling—is crucial for maintaining a healthy, positive relationship.

A wide variety of illnesses can cause or exacerbate sexual problems, but given the scope of this report, it isn't possible to include information about all of them. Here is a closer look at some of the most common culprits.

## Heart disease

Your heart is linked to your sexual organs, both physically and metaphorically. When you have chest pain or a heart attack, it's usually because fatty deposits have narrowed your arteries (a condition called atherosclerosis) and the heart tissue is not receiving enough blood. When atherosclerosis strikes the coronary arteries, it's a good bet that other vessels in your body have met the same fate—including those that serve your genitals. Because the penis needs a rapid influx of blood to achieve an erection, it's easy to see why vascular disease is the leading cause of erectile dysfunction. And for women, atherosclerosis may also cause arousal difficulties by preventing sufficient amounts of blood from reaching sex organs. Engorgement of the blood vessels of the vagina is needed for adequate lubrication and arousal.

### Medication issues

Many people with heart disease take medications to their lower blood pressure, which may cause sexual problems (see "High blood pressure," page 16). Men who take medications that contain nitrates (such as nitroglycer-

> ### ▶ Tips for resuming sex after a heart attack
> 
> Here's some advice for successful lovemaking after having a heart attack.
> - Find a time when you are both rested and relaxed. This may be in the morning or after a nap.
> - Choose a place that's comfortable and familiar, where you won't be interrupted.
> - Take any medications your health care provider may have prescribed for you to use before sex.
> - Don't feel that you need to stimulate your partner's genitals or have intercourse right away. Cuddling and caressing may be a more comfortable way to start.
> - Talk to your partner about any concerns you have. Be understanding of the emotions that both of you may be experiencing.

### Sex after a heart attack: What you need to know

If you've had a heart attack or a procedure to treat clogged arteries in your heart, how soon is it safe to have sex? Could having sex trigger another heart attack? To address these and other questions, the American Heart Association (AHA) enlisted a committee of experts to review what's known about heart disease and the safety of sex. The following Q&A features key findings from their report, which was published in 2012 in the journal *Circulation*.

**Q.** *How stressful is sex on the heart?*
**A.** Men and women have similar heart rate and blood pressure responses to sexual arousal. In young, healthy people, the physical demands of intercourse are equivalent to those of climbing two flights of stairs. In older people and people with cardiovascular disease, the effort may require greater exertion. Nevertheless, at any age, the greatest increase in heart rate and blood pressure occurs for only 10 to 15 seconds during orgasm, after which these levels quickly return to baseline.

**Q.** *What is the risk of heart attack during sex?*
**A.** Less than 1% of all heart attacks occur during sexual activity. In men, the risk is as low for those who have suffered a heart attack as it is for those without coronary artery disease. A sedentary lifestyle increases the risk, but to a much greater extent in women than in men. The good news is that having sex regularly lowers the risk, likely by improving exercise capacity.

**Q.** *What is the risk of dying during intercourse?*
**A.** Only 0.6% to 1.7% of deaths occur during intercourse, and the factors that increase risk have been clearly identified. According to the AHA report: "Of the subjects who died during coitus, 82% to 93% were men, and 75% were having extramarital sexual activity, in most cases with a younger partner in an unfamiliar setting and/or after excessive food and alcohol consumption."

**Q.** *Is sex safe after a heart attack?*
**A.** If you've had a heart attack but have no symptoms of heart disease and can pass a stress test without experiencing angina (chest pain), your risk of a heart attack during sex is low. See "Tips for resuming sex after a heart attack" on page 15 for advice.

**Q.** *When can I resume sex after an angioplasty?*
**A** Angioplasty involves threading a balloon-tipped catheter through a blood vessel to widen a narrowed artery in your heart. The site where the catheter was inserted may determine how quickly you resume sexual activity. If the procedure was done through your groin, you should wait until the puncture site has healed. If it was done through your arm, you may not need to wait any longer than a few days.

**Q.** *When can I resume sex after bypass surgery?*
**A.** After open-heart surgery to replace clogged heart arteries (bypass surgery), you should delay sexual activity until your breastbone has healed, usually six to eight weeks. For several months thereafter, avoid any position that puts stress on your chest. But if you had minimally invasive or robotic surgery, you may resume sexual activity as soon as you feel ready.

**Q.** *When is sexual activity unsafe?*
**A.** If you have unstable angina (sudden chest pain that occurs even when you are not active or stressed), worsening heart failure, uncontrolled arrhythmias (irregular heart rhythms), or severe cardiovascular disease, you should not engage in sexual activity until your condition is stable and under control.

If you experience cardiovascular symptoms during sexual activity—such as chest pain, tightness or discomfort, sweating, or shortness of breath—stop. See your health care provider, and do not resume sexual activity until your condition is stable.

**Q.** *What can I do to lower my risk?*
**A.** Although the risk of heart attack or death from sexual activity is low, you may be able to lower it further by improving your stamina. This will make the physical exertion less demanding on your heart. The best way to improve your stamina is through a cardiac rehabilitation program followed by regular, doctor-approved exercise. Exercise will also reveal how much exertion you can tolerate, which will tell you how much activity is safe for you.

---

ine) to treat angina cannot take Viagra, Levitra, or Cialis, as the interaction of nitrates with these drugs can cause a life-threatening drop in blood pressure.

## High blood pressure

Hypertension (high blood pressure), another form of vascular disease, also contributes to sexual dysfunction. It changes circulatory patterns in the body and damages the inner lining of arteries, both of which may decrease blood flow to the penis and vagina. Moreover, many popular blood pressure medications can cause erectile difficulties. In fact, sexual problems are a main reason why people stop taking drugs that lower blood pressure. But doing so can be quite dangerous, given that high blood pressure is a leading cause of stroke and also plays an important role in the physiologic changes that underlie heart attacks and heart failure.

Sexual problems attributed to high blood pressure or its treatments include impotence and ejaculation problems in men, painful or uncomfortable intercourse and difficulty having an orgasm in women, and lack of desire in both.

In theory, controlling high blood pressure should help preserve or even improve sexual function. In practice, it doesn't, at least not according to large studies. It's possible, though, that improvements in some people are offset by sexual side effects of drug therapy in others. Sexual side effects have been ascribed to virtually all classes of drugs used to control blood pressure (see Table 5, page 20). In most studies, it has been almost impossible to tell if the problem stemmed from drug therapy or high blood pressure itself. A few studies have suggested that different drug classes have different effects on sexual function, and one class—angiotensin-receptor blockers—may even improve it.

If you think a blood pressure drug is putting a damper on your sex life, talk to your health care provider, who can likely help you find a better alternative, since there are many different drugs to treat blood pressure.

## Diabetes

Unchecked, diabetes can be devastating to sexual function. About 35% to 50% of men with diabetes experience erectile dysfunction. The disease contributes to erectile problems in at least two ways: it can impair the nerves that instruct the arteries of the penis to dilate, and it can restrict blood flow to the penis by damaging the blood vessels. People with diabetes often have high blood pressure and high levels of cholesterol and other fats in the blood—all of which may further damage blood vessels and impede blood flow.

Among men with diabetes, erectile dysfunction usually develops gradually over a period of months or years. At first, the erection may not be as rigid as it once was or can't be sustained. Sometimes, erectile dysfunction is the first sign that a man has diabetes.

Carefully controlling blood sugar can help prevent the vascular and neurological complications that contribute to sexual problems. But even with proper treatment, men who have diabetes are three times as likely as other men to develop erectile dysfunction.

For women, the sexual effects of diabetes are more subtle, but they can be equally distressing. A study of more than 2,200 middle-aged and older women, published in 2012 in *Obstetrics and Gynecology*, reported lower sexual satisfaction among women who had diabetes compared with those who did not have the disease. Diabetes can damage blood vessels and nerves, interfering with clitoral sensation and vaginal lubrication and causing difficulties with arousal and orgasm. The disease may also cause low libido. In addition, high blood sugar contributes to frequent yeast and bladder infections, which can make intercourse uncomfortable for long stretches.

Many men with diabetes can take pills for erectile dysfunction, although these drugs are less effective for diabetes-related erectile dysfunction than for other causes. Studies have found that while approximately 70% of men with erectile dysfunction from other causes responded well to Viagra, only 57% of diabetic men with erectile dysfunction reported improvement. Other treatments—including drugs delivered by injection or suppository, vacuum erection devices, and penile prostheses—appear to be more helpful for diabetic men.

## Arthritis

The pain, stiffness, and flexibility problems common with arthritis often interfere with physical intimacy, especially when the hips, knees, or spine are involved. However, even people with severe arthritis can enjoy an active sex life.

A flexible attitude often compensates quite well for having a less-than-flexible body. Try different positions to find the one that is most comfortable for intercourse. For example, people with arthritis in the hips, knees, or spine often find sex most comfortable when both parties lie on their sides. Also consider expanding your sexual repertoire to include other mutually gratifying sexual activities besides intercourse.

> ### Bedtime backache?
>
> It's not uncommon for chronic back pain to interfere with lovemaking. Here are a few suggestions that may help:
>
> - Talk openly with your partner about your concerns.
> - Avoid bending your spine backward. Try to keep your spine straight or bent slightly forward.
> - When bending forward, be sure to bend your knees. Bending forward while keeping your knees straight puts a lot of pressure on your lower back.
> - Avoid lying on your stomach or your back with your legs flat on the bed and extended straight out. If you can, keep your hips flexed to take some pressure off your lower back.
> - Try positions that are easier on your back, such as lying on your side with your hips and your knees slightly bent.
> - Be judicious and gentle. If your back is bothering you, don't aim for long, vigorous, gymnastic lovemaking.
> - Making love in the water—in a pool or hot tub—can take some of the stress off your back, because water is buoyant and offers support.
> - Be patient. Don't try to resume sex too soon after having a backache. If you find that your back hurts when you resume sexual activity, wait a few days before trying again.

Rescheduling sexual activity may also help. For example, if pain and fatigue are worse in the morning, plan on a romantic afternoon instead.

Many people find that taking a painkiller—or a long, warm shower—an hour before sex eases muscle and joint stiffness. You can also place pillows under your joints to relieve pain. Special angled wedges or cushions that are designed to make intercourse more comfortable can be purchased at medical supply stores. Another option is to replace your regular bed with a waterbed.

## Cancer

The physical and psychological ramifications of cancer can deal a serious blow to sexual functioning. Cancer's effects are both direct and indirect. The disease itself can cause fatigue and pain, and the diagnosis may also engender fear, depression, guilt, stress, and poor self-image.

Cancer treatments often produce another set of problems. Nearly half of the women who undergo treatment for breast or gynecologic cancer have some long-term sexual problems. For men, prostate cancer treatment causes erectile dysfunction about 85% of the time; however, these effects vary based upon the type of treatment the man chooses. His chances of returning to sexual functioning also depend heavily on his age, his health habits, and the priority he places on sexual activity. (For one couple's perspective on dealing with these issues, see "Kate's story: Dealing with erectile dysfunction in a new relationship," page 29.) A closer look at the impact of common cancer treatments follows.

■ **Surgery.** In women, surgery that involves the pelvic organs can damage nerves, diminishing sexual sensation during intercourse. If a woman's ovaries are removed before she has reached menopause, she may experience sexual problems because of the sudden absence of estrogen as well as testosterone. Women who experience menopause at a young age due to cancer treatments, surgery, or other causes are more likely to be distressed by their sexual problems. Breast removal may deny women the pleasure of being caressed in this area, and it can have a psychological effect as well. After a mastectomy, many women struggle with body image issues and feel less sexually attractive. Most women who undergo breast reconstruction surgery note that their breast tissue is less sensitive than in the past.

For men, surgery for prostate cancer can cut nerves or arteries that are necessary for an erection. Other nerves may be damaged and need time to heal. Studies have reported that anywhere from 14% to 90% of men have erectile dysfunction after surgery to remove the prostate gland and some tissue around it (radical prostatectomy)—a range so wide that it provides little help to an individual. And even if the surgeon uses "nerve-sparing" techniques, men who do regain potency usually don't do so until about six to 12 months following surgery, though for some it can take a few years.

However, evidence suggests that using erectile dysfunction treatments right after surgery can help. When the penis is flaccid for a long period, the lack of oxygen-rich blood can cause some muscle cells in erectile tissue to lose their flexibility and gradually change into something akin to scar tissue. This seems to interfere with the penis's ability to expand. Medications called PDE5 inhibitors help dilate blood vessels and promote oxygen flow into penile tissues. One study of 22 patients found that starting sildenafil (Viagra) upon leaving the hospital after surgery, followed by penile injections several weeks later, aided the return of erections.

■ **Radiation.** Radiation treatment for prostate cancer can damage the nerves and vessels that serve the penis. It may also affect testosterone levels, leading to low libido and erection difficulties. As many as half of all men who've had this therapy have problems getting or keeping an erection. Women who have had radiation to the pelvic area can develop scar tissue in the lining of the vagina that can cause pain during intercourse. Side effects of radiation treatment—such as fatigue, nausea, vomiting, and diarrhea—are also deterrents to sexual activity.

Chemotherapy. Many of the side effects of chemotherapy, such as fatigue, nausea, hair loss, weight changes, and diarrhea, can squelch desire, damage a person's self-image, and prompt depression. Women may also notice vaginal dryness and pain. In addition, estrogen levels can drop radically during treatment, causing menopause-like symptoms. Erectile dysfunction is sometimes a side effect in men, but diminished testosterone levels and ejaculation problems are more common. Both sexes report lower sex drive and less frequent intercourse.

■ **Other treatments.** Hormone therapy for prostate cancer is aimed at reducing testosterone levels. As a result, approximately 80% of men undergoing this therapy experience low desire, erectile problems, and lack of orgasm.

The sexual effects of tamoxifen, a drug used by women to prevent breast cancer or its recurrence, are not clear. Some studies have shown that it can cause vaginal dryness or tightness, especially in postmenopausal women, while some women note an increase in lubricating vaginal secretions while taking tamoxifen.

A number of cancer treatment centers now have clinicians and even specialized clinics dedicated to sexual health and rehabilitation following cancer treatment. A 2011 article in the journal *Menopause* reported high satisfaction rates among women who received counseling and education at such a clinic based in a cancer center in Toronto.

## Depression

Depression can be both the cause and the result of sexual problems. For example, loss of desire can be a symptom of depression. Or it may appear first and provoke depression. A lack of interest in sex can lead to relationship problems, feelings of inadequacy, and other emotional issues, which in turn can result in depression. Libido isn't the only aspect of your sexuality affected by depression. Women may be less likely to have orgasms when they are depressed. And in one study, depressed men were twice as likely to experience erectile dysfunction as those who weren't depressed.

Further complicating the issue are the sexual side effects of many frequently prescribed antidepressant drugs. Medications called selective serotonin reuptake inhibitors (SSRIs)—which include fluoxetine (Prozac), sertraline (Zoloft), and paroxetine (Paxil)—can dampen desire and make it difficult to become aroused, sustain arousal, and achieve orgasm. Antidepressants can also cause vaginal dryness. An article in *Psychiatric Annals* suggests that as many as half of all people taking SSRIs experience some sexual problems.

But you don't need to sacrifice your sex life in order to treat depression. Some antidepressants—including bupropion (Wellbutrin) and mirtazapine (Remeron)—are less likely to cause sexual problems. There are reports that bupropion may boost sexual drive and arousal, as well as the intensity or duration of an orgasm, even in women without depression. Older medications, known as tricyclic antidepressants and monoamine oxidase inhibitors, don't usually cause sexual problems, but they have other numerous other unpleasant side effects. Your clinician can help you sort out which medication is right for you.

If you're taking an SSRI, taking a lower (although still therapeutic) dose may help offset or eliminate sexual problems. In the past, psychiatrists sometimes recommended taking a "drug holiday," whereby you stop taking the medication for a few days before a weekend, if that's when you hope to have sex. However, the risk that your depression may return means this practice isn't such a good idea, and the approach has fallen out of favor.

Another option is adding a drug. In both men and women, Viagra may counteract sexual problems from SSRIs. A study in *The Journal of the American Medical Association* (JAMA) found significant improvement in erectile function, arousal, ejaculation, orgasm, and overall satisfaction among men who took Viagra to counteract sexual problems stemming from SSRI use. A later JAMA study found similar results in women: nearly three of four women with sexual side effects from SSRIs who took Viagra said their sexual response improved. Yet another possible strategy is adding bupropion to your treatment for depression. You may want to ask your physician for a referral to a psychopharmacologist to help you find the best drug or drug combination for your situation.

Sex therapists offer some suggestions for coping with side effects from SSRIs, such as taking extra time to relax and spending more time stimulating the genitals before intercourse. Women might try using a vibrator, reading erotica, or masturbating beforehand, as well.

## Incontinence

Urinary incontinence (the involuntary leakage of urine) often hinders sexual function in both men and women. For women, incontinence may lower libido,

### Table 5: Medications that can cause sexual problems

| TYPE OF MEDICATION | USES | SOME EXAMPLES: GENERIC NAME (BRAND NAME) | POSSIBLE SEXUAL SIDE EFFECTS |
|---|---|---|---|
| ACE inhibitors | Heart disease | captopril (Capoten), enalapril (Vasotec), ramipril (Altace) | Low libido, erectile dysfunction |
| Antidepressants | Depression | citalopram (Celexa), fluoxetine (Prozac), paroxetine (Paxil), sertraline (Zoloft) | Low libido, erectile dysfunction, female arousal problems, orgasm difficulties |
| Antifungals | Fungal infections | amphotericin B lipid complex injection (Abelcet), itraconazole (Sporanox), ketoconazole (Nizoral) | Erectile dysfunction |
| Antihistamines | Allergies | cyproheptadine (Periactin), diphenhydramine (Benadryl), hydroxyzine (Atarax) | Vaginal dryness, erectile dysfunction |
| Anti-ulcer drugs | Acid reflux, heartburn, ulcers | cimetidine (Tagamet), famotidine (Pepcid), ranitidine (Zantac) | Low libido, erectile dysfunction |
| Beta blockers | Heart disease, high blood pressure | penbutolol (Levatol), propranolol (Inderal), timolol (Blocadren) | Low libido, erectile dysfunction, female arousal problems, orgasm difficulties |
| Calcium-channel blockers | Heart disease | diltiazem (Cardizem), nifedipine (Procardia), verapamil (Verelan) | Erectile dysfunction |
| Cholesterol-lowering drugs | High blood lipids | lovastatin (Mevacor), niacin, simvastatin (Zocor) | Erectile dysfunction |
| Diuretics | High blood pressure, fluid retention | chlorothiazide (Diuril), chlorthalidone (Thalitone), spironolactone (Aldactone) | Erectile dysfunction, female arousal problems, orgasm difficulties |
| Nitrates | Chest pain | isosorbide dinitrate (Isordil), isosorbide mononitrate (Imdur, Ismo) | Erectile dysfunction |
| Tranquilizers | Anxiety | chlordiazepoxide (Librium), diazepam (Valium), thioridazine (Mellaril) | Low libido, erectile dysfunction, female arousal problems |
| Miscellaneous | Various conditions | anti-androgens, anticholinergics, some anticancer drugs, estrogens, finasteride (Proscar and Propecia) | Erectile dysfunction |

interfere with orgasm, and contribute to pain during sex. Leaking urine during intercourse, either at penetration or during orgasm (so-called coital incontinence) affects up to about a quarter of women with incontinence, according to some estimates. But many women don't seek help for this problem, possibly because they believe it's a normal part of aging, are embarrassed, or aren't aware that effective treatments are available. However, pelvic floor muscle training, as well as surgical and medical therapies, can help—and the same is true for men with this problem, which is particularly common following prostate surgery.

## Medications

There are hundreds of potentially lifesaving medications available today to treat heart disease, depression, and a host of other problems. The downside is that some of these drugs can impair your sexual enjoyment. Table 5, page 20, lists commonly used medications that may have sexual side effects in some people. A word of caution: if you think a drug you're taking is hampering your sexual functioning, don't stop taking it without talking to your health care provider first. He or she may be able to adjust your dosage or switch you to a drug that you tolerate better.

# Treating common sexual problems

Although many adults place a high value on a healthy sex life, most don't know where to turn when sexual problems arise. Some assume that the loss of sexuality is an inevitable, although regrettable, part of aging and resign themselves to life without sex. Others are too embarrassed to seek advice, but this may only intensify feelings of frustration and inadequacy.

The popularization of Viagra in the late 1990s went a long way toward normalizing the issue of erectile dysfunction. Countless men sought help as a result. What's less well known is that many other sexual problems can also be treated effectively in men and women, often without medication.

This section describes the major types of sexual problems and provides an overview of treatment options. It's not unusual for a person to experience more than one kind of sexual problem, and therapies may overlap. Treatment often combines medication with sex therapy and self-help techniques.

### Figure 4 In working order

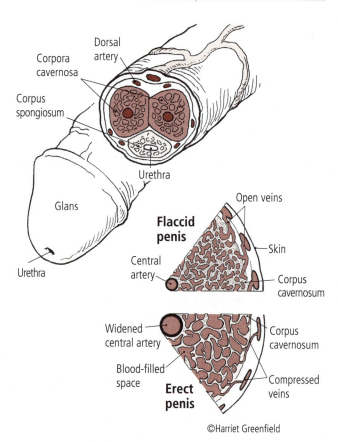

©Harriet Greenfield

When a man is sexually stimulated, chemical signals from the brain cause the penile arteries to widen, allowing more blood to enter the erectile bodies known as the corpora cavernosa. The tissues swell with blood, causing an erection. At the same time, the blood-engorged tissues compress the veins, keeping blood in the penis and maintaining the erection.

## Erectile dysfunction

Although erectile dysfunction becomes more common as men age, this problem isn't an inevitable part of aging. While age-related changes such as lower testosterone levels, decreased blood flow to the genitals, slower nerve function, less elastic erectile tissue, and increased stress all play a part, even these factors don't fully explain all the numbers. The problem often results from an illness that becomes more prevalent with age—such as cardiovascular disease or diabetes—or its treatment. Many of these conditions can be prevented with good health habits such as following a healthy diet, exercising regularly, maintaining a normal weight, and not smoking.

### How an erection occurs

At its most basic level, an erection is a hydraulic event. Blood fills the penis, causing it to swell and become firm. But getting to that stage requires an extraordinary orchestration of body mechanisms. Most of the time, an erection really starts in the man's brain. A sight, smell, or touch sparks electrical signals of sexual arousal in the brain. These signals travel from the brain to an area in the lower part of the spinal cord. Nerves in this area signal nerves in the pelvis, which instruct arteries to let blood into the penis, thereby causing an erection (see Figure 4, at left).

## Causes of erectile dysfunction

In the past, most cases of erectile dysfunction were considered psychological, the result of such demons as performance anxiety or more general stress. Although these factors do cause some cases of erectile dysfunction, experts think that 70% of cases can be traced to age-related changes or a physical condition that hampers blood flow, nerve functioning, or both. Such conditions include diabetes, kidney disease, atherosclerosis, vascular disease, multiple sclerosis, and alcoholism (see "Health problems and sexuality," page 15). Less frequently, erectile dysfunction is an outgrowth of injury to the nerves and vessels that serve the genitals or a disease that causes scarring of penile tissue.

Unhealthy habits can also raise a man's risk of erectile dysfunction. A study in *The Journal of Urology* showed that smoking raises the risk of erectile dysfunction by 50%, while being obese increases risk by 90%. Men who were both overweight and sedentary were two-and-a-half times as likely to have erectile dysfunction as were active men of normal weight.

But thinking of erectile dysfunction as either psychological or physical can be misleading. These forces are usually intertwined. In fact, more than 80% of men with erectile dysfunction caused by an underlying physical illness develop psychological issues that further hamper erections.

## Diagnosing the problem

Before going to your clinician, it's important to understand what erectile dysfunction really is. Failure to get an erection after one too many drinks or during a week of intense stress doesn't constitute erectile dysfunction. Also, normal changes in your sexual response as you age—such as having to wait a longer time after orgasm to have another erection or needing more direct stimulation—don't necessarily fall under this heading.

Erectile dysfunction is the inability to attain and maintain an erection sufficient for sexual intercourse at least 25% of the time. The penis doesn't get hard enough, or it gets hard but softens too soon. The problem generally comes on gradually. When such difficulties occur regularly and distress you or your partner, it's time to talk to your health care provider.

He or she will ask about your symptoms and your health history, including any diseases and surgeries you've had and medications you're taking. Other queries may address feelings of depression, your stress level, and your relationship with your partner. Sometimes, having your partner come to your doctor's appointment can be helpful, although some men may prefer to go alone (see "Advice for partners," below).

During an exam, the clinician will check for conditions that can affect blood flow, such as high blood pressure or a heart murmur. He or she may test your blood to assess your risk for cardiovascular disease.

### ▶ Advice for partners

A man with erectile dysfunction isn't the only one who's affected by it; the impact extends to his partner as well. As his partner, you may want to help but not know how. Here are suggestions for some things you can do.

**Discuss the issue.** Good communication is the foundation of an enduring relationship. Confront any concerns you may have about erectile difficulties by discussing your feelings and telling your partner that you care. Often it's best to talk at a time and place where both people will feel less vulnerable—that is, not while in bed with your clothes off.

**Reassure your partner that he is not alone.** Remind him (and yourself) that millions of men have erectile dysfunction and that it's a treatable medical condition.

**Learn about the condition and treatment options.** Information truly is empowering. The best treatment for erectile dysfunction is one that you both agree will fit most comfortably with your lovemaking.

**Offer to go with your partner to his appointment.** In general, couples who work together have the best chance of successful treatment. But if your partner prefers to see his clinician alone, respect his privacy. There are other ways you can support his treatment.

**Help your partner help himself.** Keep in mind that bad health habits, such as smoking and heavy drinking, can cause erectile dysfunction. In a supportive and nonjudgmental way, encourage your partner to break these habits. What's good for his overall health is good for your sexual relationship.

**Express your love in many ways.** Expand your repertoire of intimate expressions. Lovemaking can be satisfying even without an erection.

The clinician will also examine your testicles, penis, and chest (small testicles and enlarged breasts are signs of low testosterone). In addition, he or she will feel your prostate gland and test your reflexes. Now that medication can successfully treat most cases of erectile dysfunction, many once-routine diagnostic tests are rarely used. Still, if your clinician suspects that you have another condition that requires treatment, he or she may order a specialized test.

## Treatments for erectile dysfunction

Health care providers can choose from a number of options for treating erectile dysfunction, including some that don't involve any drugs or devices (see "Six all-natural sex tips," below). Table 6, page 26, compares the other options, which range from the well-known PDE5 inhibitor drugs such as Viagra to lesser-known treatments such as injections, pellets, pumps, and bands, which are also described below.

In rare cases, when no other options succeed, surgery may be an option (see "Surgical implants," page 25).

■ **The PDE5 inhibitors:** Viagra, Levitra, and Cialis. When sildenafil (Viagra) came onto the market in the late 1990s, it revolutionized the treatment of erectile dysfunction. The famous "little blue pill" is safe, easy to use, and effective for a broad range of causes—qualities that made it the first-line treatment for most men with erectile dysfunction. Its success spawned competitors like vardenafil (Levitra) and tadalafil (Cialis), both of which were approved by the FDA in 2003.

All three medications work in much the same way: by relaxing smooth muscle cells, the drugs widen blood vessels primarily in the penis, as well as in other parts of the body. For many men, this clears the way for an erection. These pills aren't aphrodisiacs; you've got to feel desire and be sexually stimulated in order for them to work. But if they are taken 15 minutes to an hour before intercourse, they can help you get and

### Six all-natural sex tips

Looking for natural ways to sidestep or help reverse erectile dysfunction? Skip the supplements and try these tips for a better sex life and general health. Improved mood and quality of life are added bonuses.

1. **Start walking.** Just 30 minutes of walking a day was linked with a 41% drop in risk for erectile dysfunction, according to one Harvard study, while a separate trial reported that moderate exercise can help restore sexual performance in obese middle-aged men with erectile dysfunction.

2. **Eat right.** Go bullish on fruit, vegetables, whole grains, and fish, while downplaying red and processed meat and refined grains, a diet that lessened the likelihood of erectile dysfunction in the Massachusetts Male Aging Study. Another tip: chronic deficiencies in vitamin $B_{12}$—found in clams, salmon, trout, beef, fortified cereals, and yogurt—may harm the spinal cord, potentially short-circuiting nerves responsible for sensation as well as for relaying messages to arteries in the penis. Multivitamins and fortified foods are the best bets for people who absorb $B_{12}$ poorly, including many older adults and anyone with atrophic gastritis, a condition that may affect nearly one in three people ages 50 and older.

3. **Check your vascular health.** Signs that put you on the road to poor vascular health include soaring levels of blood pressure, blood sugar, LDL (bad) cholesterol, and triglycerides; low levels of HDL (good) cholesterol; and a widening waist. Check with your clinician to find out whether your vascular system—and thus your heart, brain, and penis—is in good shape or needs a tune-up through lifestyle changes and, if necessary, medications.

4. **Measure up.** A trim waistline is one good defense—a man with a 42-inch waist is 50% more likely to have erectile dysfunction than one with a 32-inch waist.

5. **Slim down.** Tip the scales at a healthy weight. Obesity raises risks for vascular disease and diabetes, two major causes of erectile dysfunction. And excess fat tinkers with several hormones that may feed into the problem, too. Need more reasons? Slimming down helps with tips 3 and 4.

6. **Move a muscle.** Actually, move several muscles of the pelvic floor, including the ischiocavernosus, which enhances rigidity during erections, and the bulbocavernosus, which helps keep blood from leaving the penis by pressing on a key vein. In a randomized, controlled trial of 55 British men, three months of twice-daily sets of Kegel exercises, which strengthen these muscles, combined with biofeedback plus advice on lifestyle changes—quitting smoking, losing weight, limiting alcohol—worked far better than just advice on lifestyle changes. During the next three months, the control group also practiced Kegels and experienced similar improvements in erections. At six months, 40% of all the subjects had regained normal erectile function, and an additional nearly 36% had improved.

maintain an erection by acting on the normal physiology of the penis.

The three medications have similar success rates. In all, about 70% of men respond well to the drugs, but the rates vary according to what is responsible for the erectile dysfunction. Men with impotence of no identifiable physical cause fare best, while the drugs are less effective for men with diabetes or who have had prostate cancer surgery.

Despite their impressive results, these medications have some drawbacks. Since they can take up to an hour to work, you'll need to plan accordingly. Some insurance plans do not cover these drugs, and others allow for only a few pills a month. Even if you don't think you'll use all the pills allotted to you each month, you might consider ordering them anyway, so that you'll have extras on hand for vacations or special occasions.

Men who take nitrates (such as nitroglycerin tablets, cream, or patches) cannot take PD5 inhibitors, as this combination can cause dangerously low blood pressure. Men with unstable cardiovascular disease also should avoid Viagra and related drugs.

■ **Yohimbine.** This plant-based remedy is extracted from the bark of the yohimbe tree. Studies of its effectiveness have been inconsistent, and clinicians don't recommend it as a first-line therapy. However, it may be useful for men who are unable to take PDE5 inhibitors. Side effects include insomnia, increased heart rate and blood pressure, nervousness, irritability, and dizziness. For more on yohimbine, see "Alternative therapies for sexual problems" on page 37.

■ **Penile injections.** For men who can't or don't want to use PDE5 inhibitors, injecting medication directly into the side of the penis with a tiny needle is an effective option. Injection therapy works better than erectile dysfunction pills for men whose erectile difficulties result from diabetes or prostate cancer surgery. Men with diabetes often report that the penile

> ### Surgical implants
> 
> This option is reserved for cases where no other form of treatment has succeeded. Two kinds of implants are available. The first consists of two pencil-thin silicone rods implanted in the penile shaft above the urethra. The operation is done on an outpatient basis and takes about an hour. Afterward, the penis remains permanently erect, although it can be pointed down along the thigh to conceal it under clothing.
> 
> The second type of implant uses inflatable cylinders that are placed into the corpora cavernosa. When the man wants an erection, he simply squeezes a pump located in the scrotum. The pump pushes saline fluid into the cylinders from a reservoir implanted in the scrotum or abdomen. Although this device generates a more natural erection than silicone rods, it's prone to complications, such as infection or malfunction.

### Safer sex and erectile dysfunction

Passing your 50th birthday does not guarantee immunity from sexually transmitted infections (STIs). The rate of STIs has more than doubled among middle-aged adults and the elderly over the last decade. Therefore, if you find yourself contemplating a new sexual relationship after a long stretch of being with the same partner or sexual inactivity, you may be faced with taking safer sex precautions for the first time. Primary among these is the use of a condom during sex, which many older people often don't consider because they're not worried about pregnancy.

Safe sex is especially important for postmenopausal women because they are more vulnerable to STIs than younger women, for several reasons. As estrogen levels drop off after menopause, the vaginal and cervical tissues thin. This condition, called vaginal atrophy, makes the vaginal lining vulnerable to small tears and abrasions, which provide points of entry for viruses and bacteria. In addition, age-related decline in immune response may make it harder to fight off an STI. And STIs in older women may go undetected because they often have no symptoms, and clinicians aren't always tuned in to screening older women.

Many men who have had a history of erectile difficulties may balk at the thought of using a condom for fear that a break in the action will cause them to lose their erection. Here are some tips for how you can avoid erection problems while still playing it safe:

• Have the condom unwrapped and within easy reach.

• Let your partner help you put the condom on if that person is comfortable doing so.

• Focus on an erotic fantasy while you put on the condom. This will keep you from worrying about your erection.

• Stimulate your penis as you get the condom ready and slip it on.

injections hurt no more than insulin shots. Your health care provider can demonstrate the injection technique, which most men are able to learn quickly. Only one drug, alprostadil (Caverject and Edex), is approved specifically to treat erectile dysfunction in this manner, although several older drugs used for other purposes are also effective. These include papaverine (Pavabid, Genabid, and others), phenoxybenzamine (Dibenzyline), and phentolamine (Regitine).

■ **Drug pellets and MUSE.** An alternative to injections is a therapy called MUSE (which stands for "medicated urethral system for erection"). In this procedure, you use a disposable plastic applicator to insert a pellet of the drug alprostadil (the same drug that's used in injections) about an inch up the urethra. From there the drug is quickly absorbed into the erectile tissues, where it dilates the arteries. Some men find it easier to use than injections.

■ **Mechanical devices.** Men who can't or don't want to use medications can opt for mechanical devices that assist in producing an erection, maintaining an erection, or both.

### Table 6: Comparing treatments for erectile dysfunction (ED)

| THERAPY | HOW SOON IT STARTS TO WORK | HOW LONG IT LASTS | ADVANTAGES | DISADVANTAGES | APPROXIMATE COST |
|---|---|---|---|---|---|
| sildenafil (Viagra) | 30–60 minutes | 4–5 hours | Oral medication, very effective (about 70%), few side effects | Cannot be used by men taking nitrates or those with unstable cardiovascular disease | About $15–$20 per dose |
| vardenafil (Levitra) | 15–30 minutes | 4–5 hours | | | |
| tadalafil (36-hour Cialis) | 30–45 minutes | 24–36 hours | | | |
| tadalafil (Cialis for daily use) | Ongoing | Anytime sexual arousal occurs | Oral medication. According to one small study, effectiveness varies depending on dose (2.5 mg or 5 mg) and level of ED, ranging from 27% for severe ED to 82% for mild ED. | Same as above | About $4–$5 per day |
| yohimbine (Yocon) | 2–3 weeks with daily use | As long as therapy continues | Oral medication; somewhat effective (40%); a good option for men who cannot use Viagra and related drugs | Side effects include insomnia, increased heart rate and blood pressure, nervousness | About $0.27–$0.54 per day |
| alprostadil injections (Caverject, Edex) | 5–20 minutes | 30–60 minutes | Highly effective (about 80%); few side effects | Requires training; injections unpleasant for many men; may cause penile pain or painful sustained erections | $43–$49 per dose |
| alprostadil pellets (MUSE) | 5–15 minutes | 30–60 minutes | Moderately effective (about 30%) | Requires training; may cause penile pain, usually mild; may cause dizziness | $30–$36 per use |
| vacuum pump | Immediate | Until the band placed at base of penis after using the vacuum pump is removed | Highly effective (about 80%); no serious side effects | Requires training; cumbersome and awkward; may cause penile numbness or bruising | $160–$425 per device (a one-time cost) |
| penile band (Actis, Erecxel) | Immediate | While in use | Effective when used properly; helpful for men with venous leakage who cannot sustain an erection | May be awkward to use | $4–$16 per band (reusable) |

- **Vacuum pump.** This device consists of an airtight plastic cylinder that's attached to a manual or battery-operated handheld pump. You insert your penis into the cylinder and pump out the air, which increases blood flow to the penis. It takes about five minutes to get an erection. At that point, you fit a rubber ring around the base of the penis to prevent the blood from draining away. The erection lasts until the ring is removed. Some men find the pump hard to use, the process may be disruptive to lovemaking, and the man's erection does not feel as natural as one produced with medication. But the device is very effective and causes no side effects.
- **Penile band.** If you can get an erection but lose it because of leakage of blood from veins in the penis, you may find a penile band helpful. This band is fastened around the base of the penis to prevent blood from escaping. Available without a prescription under the brand names Actis and Erecxel, the bands are very effective when used properly.

### How sex therapy can help

Sex therapy is often helpful for erectile dysfunction, even when physical factors are the principal cause. Sexual difficulties, no matter what their origin, can strain your relationship. Frequently a man with erectile problems experiences performance anxiety, which makes him reluctant to initiate sexual contact. His partner may perceive this as rejection or lack of attraction, which could trigger feelings of frustration, insecurity, and resentment. Sex therapy can help a couple overcome these feelings and re-establish intimacy.

In addition to standard sensate focus techniques (see page 42), the therapist may teach the couple mindfulness techniques that aim to keep them focused on the present moment, which can help overcome worries about losing an erection during sexual activity.

Another suggestion for couples to practice at home is for a man and his partner to progress to the stage of sexual excitement and stimulation where intercourse would normally begin, then to purposely stop so that the penis becomes less firm. Then they resume stimulation until the man has an erection again. When they do this exercise repeatedly, the couple usually learns to relax, focus on the sensations and pleasure, recognizing that the man will often be able to regain his erection again if he loses it.

It's common for sex therapy to be used along with medications for erectile dysfunction. Clinicians often prescribe drugs to help men overcome performance anxiety in the short term and recommend sex therapy to help the couple work through the emotional component of the problem. Once confidence is restored, some men are able to have erections without taking Viagra or similar medications.

## Low libido

Diminished sex drive is the most common and the most elusive sexual dysfunction. According to a 1994 landmark study of sexuality in America conducted by University of Chicago researchers, 33% of women and 16% of men reported they had gone through periods of several months when they had no interest in sex. A particularly challenging aspect of the problem is that it often exists along with one or more other sexual dysfunctions. For example, a woman who experiences painful intercourse will understandably shy away from sexual activity.

### What is desire?

To determine what constitutes low libido, it's important to first understand the nature of desire. The three main aspects of desire are sexual drive, sexual wish, and sexual motive. Sexual drive is a hormone-dependent impulse for sexual release. It can manifest itself as a longing to reproduce or to have sex, erotic thoughts or dreams, or an urge to masturbate. Sexual wish is the willingness to have sex. Even if an individual's physiological need for sex is weak, he or she may wish to participate in the activity to feel more connected to another person, to feel more masculine or feminine, or to feel more emotionally alive and physically energetic. Sexual motive is the combination of factors that impel a person to want sex. All three of these elements have to be taken into account when examining libido problems. Of all the forms of sexual dysfunction, low desire is the most complex and challenging to treat.

The diagnosis of low libido is quite subjective. There are no physical signs to measure, and the level of libido varies widely from person to person. Age, sex, personality, stage of life, physical and psychological health, and the relationship with the partner all play a role. Medically, low libido is defined as the absence of sexual fantasies or a lack of desire for sexual activity that causes personal distress. However, this too can vary. Because there's a range of desire levels within "normal" libido, significant differences in the level of sexual interest can create tension in a relationship. If the person with lower desire is strongly pressured to have sex, this can further reduce his or her sexual interest.

To complicate matters, female desire has been historically misunderstood. Researchers have questioned the assumption that libido manifests itself in the same way in women as in men. They propose that while men's desire is driven by the goal of intercourse and orgasm, women's desire is often driven by the need for intimacy. In addition, some women may need to be physically aroused before feeling desire.

Age is also a factor, as desire tends to wane with age. It can flag in midlife for a variety of reasons—some physical, some emotional. Hallmarks of aging such as hormonal declines or lifestyle and relationship transitions can all affect a person's sex drive. So too can illness and the presence of other sexual problems, such as erectile dysfunction or vaginal dryness and discomfort. Of course, if a lower sex drive isn't bothersome to the people involved, then they need not take any action. If diminished sex drive is troublesome, though, treatment is available.

### Diagnosing low libido

When evaluating a loss of sexual desire, your health care provider will first look for physical causes. Any of a number of chronic medical conditions can impinge on desire (see "Health problems and sexuality," page 15). So, too, can treatments for these conditions, including a wide variety of medications and procedures. The emotional effects of almost any chronic disease—such as frustration, depression, anger, fear of death, and altered body image—can indirectly lead to the loss of desire. In women, low libido may also stem from chronic vaginal, vulvar, or pelvic pain, which will typically cause discomfort with intercourse.

If there are no obvious physical reasons for low libido, your clinician will explore your sexual history, including your attitudes and feelings about sex and your relationship with your partner. One important distinction to be made is whether the problem is a lifelong lack of desire, a more recent loss of interest, or a problem that occurs only with a particular partner or in a certain situation. Sometimes, a history of physical or sexual abuse can manifest as low libido (or an aversion to sex) that may not show up until after the person has married or had children (see "Coping with a history of sexual abuse," page 35).

If your libido has dropped significantly, your clinician will focus on the point when the change occurred and explore potential physiological and emotional causes. He or she will ask about symptoms stemming from menopause or aging and ask about your relationship with your partner. The provider will also ask about your levels of stress and fatigue, self-image, and whether depression may be a factor.

### Treating the problem

If a medication is contributing to the problem, your clinician may suggest switching to a new drug or lowering your dose. While hormone changes are sometimes involved, often the problem stems from a mix of physiological, psychological, and relationship issues. If, after careful questioning and a physical exam, your clinician decides that the problem would improve with nonmedical treatment, many options are available, from stress reduction to sex therapy and relationship-building strategies.

■ **Sex therapy.** Low libido is the most common, challenging, and complex problem a sex therapist encounters. An early obstacle is that individuals with low libido often aren't eager to be treated—because they don't miss sex, because they don't feel hopeful about finding a solution, or because they worry that there is something seriously wrong with them or with the relationship. Most of the time they consent to therapy when they feel the problem is threatening their relationship.

Therapists often address this issue in a variety of ways. Usually, the problem is recast as a couples issue; therapy isn't a means to "cure" the person with the low sex drive. The therapist aims to reassure the low-

## Kate's story: Dealing with erectile dysfunction in a new relationship

*Sexual problems can be challenging for couples who have been together for a long time, but a shared history can sometimes make talking about the problem a little easier. Single middle-aged and older adults don't have that advantage, and new relationships can be tricky to navigate for a variety of reasons. The following story describes how one new couple successfully dealt with erectile dysfunction that resulted from prostate cancer surgery. The couples' names have been changed.*

Kate, age 48, met her boyfriend, David, age 54, at a friend's Thanksgiving dinner. The two had an almost instant connection and started dating. Because they spent so much time talking about their lives and discovering all that they had in common, they quickly grew close. So Kate didn't find it odd when David told her on their first date that he had been treated for prostate cancer four years earlier.

"I told him that my mother was about to have a mastectomy, and he said that he had been through prostate cancer," she recalls. "Maybe it was a little early in the relationship, but he was so matter-of-fact about it and needed so little prompting that it wasn't an uncomfortable discussion at all. So, I knew before our first sexual encounter and didn't think twice about it."

David revealed that he opted to have his prostate removed. The cancer, which was detected through screening, was small, and its location meant that the nerve bundles could be left intact. After the operation, he suffered from incontinence for a few months, and he had to wear a pad when he went running. He also started taking tadalafil, but after a few months, that wasn't necessary. He could have an erection without it.

"He also told me that he has a dry orgasm. It never occurred to me that a man would not ejaculate after prostate surgery, but I thought it was wonderful," says Kate with a laugh. "He was the perfect man. No cleanup would be necessary, and I wouldn't have to reach for the box of tissues afterward!"

Her sense of humor probably helped ease any tension after they tried to have intercourse for the first time. "Even though he said that he'd never had a problem before, he wasn't able to sustain an erection with me. I didn't know what to think because he seemed so aroused. But he also seemed frustrated and unnerved. He kept saying he wanted to share that experience with me, and he seemed genuinely surprised by his inability to stay hard."

More attempts at intercourse, all unsuccessful, followed. "I thought he was putting too much pressure on himself and that it was just performance anxiety," says Kate. "I also started thinking that maybe he still had feelings for a previous partner, but he said that wasn't it. And he said I must have thought he was lying to me about his ability to have an erection.

"In retrospect, there was probably too much focus on the lack of an erection and orgasm," says Kate. "I reassured him that I was enjoying the intimacy we had together. He was enjoying my orgasms if not his own!"

David decided to try taking tadalafil again, because he responded well to it in the months after his surgery. It worked. "After that first success, it was sheer relief for him," says Kate. "I think he felt the need to prove himself and to show that he was still young, sexy, and capable. The sexual piece is part of his identity.

"After we 'accomplished the mission,' he thanked me for my patience. That made me realize that he thought I might give up on the relationship, but I honestly never considered that. I certainly would've felt that I was missing out on something if there wasn't any physical intimacy; I think that's an integral part of a relationship. But his having an erection wasn't a 'make or break' for me."

Kate wonders whether David will continue with the tadalafil regularly if he needs to—she wants him to but is afraid to ask. She doesn't want him to think she wouldn't stay with him if he stops taking it. "It's difficult because the relationship is so new, and we're both finding our way. It is a sensitive subject, but this will be a good test of how we communicate about all kinds of things," she says.

---

desire partner that he or she won't be forced or even pressured by the therapist to have sex. The therapist will explore whether the individual may be missing out on a valuable part of life (and a way of being closer with a partner). The therapist also works to diminish any pent-up resentment on the part of the higher-drive partner by noting that he or she is making a choice to stay committed to the relationship by engaging in the search for a joint solution. The goal of treatment is to help create an atmosphere in the relationship that is less pressured, thereby allowing the low-desire partner to become more receptive to feeling and being sexual.

Another important step is to have the partner with the lower libido recognize, explore, and come to terms with any hidden feelings of anger, resentment, guilt, fear, or disgust that surround sex. If these feelings are present, the couple and the therapist explore the origins and impact of these emotions. This may take multiple sessions. The therapist may also gently challenge the couple's assumptions about how sex "should be." Sometimes sex can just be good enough. It doesn't always have to be spontaneous, creative, passionate, and satisfying for both members of the couple. The therapist will encourage the couple to examine the dynamics of the relationship that reinforce the discrepancy in desire. For example, the bedroom may be a venue for acting out power struggles, with the person who otherwise feels ineffectual in the relationship unconsciously avoiding sex as a means of control.

### Testosterone for women

When it comes to hormone therapy, estrogen gets all the attention. But testosterone is also a key player in a woman's sexual response, and testosterone therapy is occasionally used as a way to treat low sexual desire associated with distress in postmenopausal women.

Testosterone production peaks in a woman's 20s and gradually declines after that. By menopause, it registers at just about half of what it was at its peak. The hormone doesn't disappear completely, however. The ovaries manufacture it throughout life, even though they stop producing estrogen at menopause. But if a woman's ovaries are removed (which sometimes occurs in combination with a hysterectomy), her testosterone levels drop, although the adrenal glands continue to make hormones similar to testosterone. The same decline can occur after certain forms of chemotherapy.

Taking oral estrogen can also diminish a woman's testosterone levels, because her body responds to the increased amount of estrogen by boosting its production of a protein known as SHBG. This protein binds to testosterone, so other cells in the body cannot then use the testosterone.

Although testosterone may influence certain aspects of sexual response, large studies in women of all ages have not identified a clear link between testosterone levels and sexual desire and satisfaction. What is the role of testosterone in female sexuality? Researchers are still exploring the answer to this question. Although the medical community has long been aware of the role of so-called male hormones in women's sexuality, testosterone therapy remains controversial, and no testosterone products are yet FDA-approved for use in women.

Several studies have found that skin patches that deliver 300 micrograms of testosterone daily can boost sexual desire and the number of satisfying sexual encounters in women with distressing low desire who have gone through menopause (either naturally or from surgery to remove their ovaries). It's important to realize that all of the women who participated in these studies had no other potential cause for their low libido. They were physically and psychologically healthy, were not using antidepressants or other medications that could affect sexual function, and were in long-term sexual relationships they described as caring and communicative. These studies, most of which lasted six months, found only minor side effects from the hormone, including mild acne, increased facial hair, and skin irritation under the patch. The patches used in these studies are not approved for use in the United States, as the FDA is waiting for more safety data. A long-term study of a testosterone gel should provide information soon on whether testosterone increases the risk of heart disease or breast cancer in women. Interestingly, although this testosterone gel product increases testosterone blood levels to the same degree as did the testosterone patches, a recent study showed that the testosterone gel was no more effective in increasing libido and sexual response than a placebo gel.

Some clinicians are prescribing specially formulated testosterone lotions and gels for women, but the quality and dose of these compounded products, which are made to order at special pharmacies, are inconsistent. In women, side effects can include acne, liver problems, and a slight drop in HDL (good) cholesterol, as well as a deeper voice and facial and body hair. Women who use testosterone therapy should have their blood testosterone levels checked periodically to ensure they don't get too high.

Testosterone is converted to estrogen in the blood, and some experts are concerned that the risks of estrogen therapy, such as breast cancer, heart disease, and stroke, will also be seen in women on testosterone therapy. In fact, one study found that the risk of breast cancer was nearly 2.5 times greater in postmenopausal women who took hormone pills combining estrogen and testosterone than in those who didn't take the medications. The researchers also reported that the risk of breast cancer was greater with estrogen-testosterone therapy than with estrogen alone or estrogen combined with progesterone. One study on testosterone patches, published in 2008 in the *New England Journal of Medicine*, documented four cases of breast cancer among women using the patches, but no cases in the placebo group—a difference that could be due to chance but is worrisome nonetheless. Clearly, more study is needed to determine how testosterone might influence the risk of breast cancer.

Over-the-counter DHEA (dehydroepiandrosterone) supplements are promoted as another way to help produce testosterone in the body. There's little reliable evidence that they reduce menopausal symptoms or improve sexual function in healthy women. In one study, published in 2009 in *The Journal of Sexual Medicine*, researchers gave 93 postmenopausal women with low libido either 50 milligrams of DHEA or a placebo daily. After six months, they found no difference in satisfying sexual experiences or well-being between the two groups.

However, a vaginal form of DHEA has shown some promise. Early reports suggest that postmenopausal women who use a nightly DHEA vaginal suppository report less vaginal dryness, more sexual arousal and lubrication, and some improvement in orgasm. Further studies are under way.

Once most of the emotional and attitudinal roadblocks have been addressed, the couple moves on to behavioral exercises designed to increase trust, communication, and sensual awareness (see "Sensate focus," page 42). This can help the couple begin to slowly re-establish physical intimacy. When a person's low desire is an outgrowth of a sexual problem within the relationship, treatment for low desire is usually an easier matter once the original sexual difficulty is resolved.

**Medical treatments.** Medical treatments for libido problems are often combined with sex therapy. The following options are available:

- **Hormone treatment for men.** Although there's a clear link between testosterone production and male libido, researchers have yet to discover the exact nature of the connection. If a man's hormone level is clearly below normal, testosterone supplements can make a noticeable difference in his libido. On the other hand, supplements seem to have no effect on men whose natural testosterone is already within a normal range. The impact of testosterone supplements on men who have borderline or low-normal hormone levels is still unknown. Although desire wanes with age, this problem doesn't seem to be linked to declining testosterone (see "Testing testosterone," page 6).

- **Hormone treatment for women.** Many people don't realize that women also produce testosterone naturally, and this hormone affects libido in women as it does in men, although the connection is less clear. The natural decline of testosterone that accompanies aging may affect a woman's sexual interest and responsiveness. As a result, some health care providers prescribe testosterone, although information on its safety and effectiveness is limited (see "Testosterone for women," page 30).

- **Bupropion.** This antidepressant may increase sexual desire and arousal in men and women without depression, in addition to countering the negative sexual side effects of SSRI antidepressant medications in those with depression, according to several studies. People who take SSRIs, such as citalopram (Celexa), fluoxetine (Prozac), paroxetine (Paxil), and sertraline (Zoloft), may want to ask their clinicians about trying bupropion instead of, or in addition to, their SSRI.

# Female sexual arousal disorder

When a woman becomes aroused through thoughts and fantasies, physical stimulation, or both, blood flows to her pelvic region, causing her genital tissues to swell and her vagina to moisten (see "The phases of sexual response," page 3). These changes indicate the beginning of her physical readiness for sexual activity. With female sexual arousal disorder, however, the sequence breaks down. A woman may be distressed if her body doesn't produce this response, or if it occurs but doesn't correspond to her emotional state. Interestingly, studies that use probes to measure genital swelling confirm that there is often a disconnect between physiological arousal and a woman's awareness of these changes.

### Making a diagnosis

Your health care provider will first want to hear your account of any problems you have becoming aroused and achieving and maintaining vaginal lubrication in response to sexual excitement. He or she may ask detailed questions about your general physical and emotional health, the stresses in your life, your relationship with your partner, your expectations about sex based on your upbringing, and the amount of foreplay and direct stimulation you receive during lovemaking, as well as all the medications you're taking. It's particularly important to consider whether you've gone through menopause, as the drop in estrogen that occurs at menopause can cause vaginal atrophy, in which the tissue thins and secretions decrease. Over time, especially if intercourse is infrequent, the vagina and vaginal opening narrow. Intercourse then becomes painful, resulting in decreased libido and arousal. It's likely that your clinician will also perform a pelvic exam.

### Increasing genital blood flow

Speculation that women's arousal difficulties may be related to insufficient blood flow opened a possible avenue of treatment for female sexual arousal disorder. But efforts to find a female Viagra haven't panned out thus far. Pfizer, the company that makes Viagra, tested the drug in women for eight years. Studies found that the drug increased genital blood flow, but for most women that didn't translate into more sexual arousal or a greater desire to have sex. Still, other researchers and companies are studying and selling products aimed at increasing genital blood flow in women. Here's a closer look at a few of them.

■ **Topical medications.** Researchers are studying several creams and gels that deliver medication to widen blood vessels. These products are rubbed into the genital tissues before intercourse to enhance arousal. Compounds effective in men, including prostaglandin E-1 and phentolamine, have been tested in women but are still considered experimental. Additionally, the over-the-counter supplement Zestra claims to enhance sexual function in part by increasing genital blood flow (see "Alternative therapies for sexual problems," page 37).

■ **Mechanical devices.** A small pumplike device—consisting of a plastic cup that fits over the clitoris and surrounding tissue—uses suction to draw blood into the clitoris, causing it to swell. This FDA-approved unit is sold by prescription to women with arousal disorders under the brand name Eros-CTD (clitoral therapy device). However, such devices are costly and rarely covered by insurance. A less expensive option is to try a vibrator, which can also increase blood flow.

## Treating vaginal dryness

Vaginal dryness is a common cause of female sexual arousal disorder and can also contribute to low libido. A reduction or absence of lubrication and the related loss of elasticity can make intercourse uncomfortable. Several different treatments are available, ranging from over-the-counter lubricants to prescription hormone treatments. For many women, lubricants and vaginal moisturizers will do the trick, so they're a good place to start. If these products aren't helpful, low-dose vaginal estrogen products—available as creams, tablets, or rings inserted into the vagina—can raise estrogen levels in the vagina, making the tissue thicker and more elastic. Because blood levels of estrogen are not significantly increased with low-dose vaginal estrogen formulations, these products are very safe and not associated with the risks seen with higher-dose estrogen therapy, which boosts estrogen levels throughout the body. Still, higher-dose estrogen therapy—available as pills, patches, gels, sprays, or rings—remains an option for women who experience other uncomfortable symptoms during menopause, such as hot flashes, night sweats, and insomnia, in addition to vaginal symptoms. Below is an overview of the various choices. Table 7, below, lists the different types of low-dose vaginal estrogen therapy, and Table 8 on page 33, lists the different types of higher-dose estrogen therapy.

■ **Vaginal lubricants.** If vaginal dryness with sexual activity is your primary or only concern, a lubricating liquid or gel that temporarily alleviates vaginal discomfort with sex may be your best solution. One example is Astroglide, a clear, thin, odorless liquid with a slippery feel that closely approximates natural vaginal secretions. You can apply it to the vaginal opening or to the penis before intercourse. This water-based product is nonstaining and has a neutral pH, so it won't irritate the vagina or promote vaginal infections. K-Y Sensual Silk and related K-Y products offer similar benefits. Vaginal lubricants can increase sexual pleasure, and you may wish to try several different products to find the one you and your partner prefer.

■ **Long-acting vaginal moisturizers.** These products are very effective at treating vaginal dryness when placed in the vagina several nights a week on a regular basis. They cling to the vaginal lining, helping to retain moisture, similar to moisturizers you use on your hands or face. One example, Replens, is inserted into the vagina with an applicator and lasts up to three days. A related product, K-Y Liquibeads, consists of small beads that are also inserted with an applicator and last up to four days. These products are a good option if your dryness is bothersome even when you're not engaged

### Table 7: Low-dose vaginal estrogen therapy for vaginal atrophy

These products, which contain low doses of hormones, can reverse tissue thinning, dryness, and other age-related changes of the vagina.

| Hormone(s) | Trade name | How taken? |
|---|---|---|
| Estradiol and conjugated estrogens | Estrace vaginal cream, Premarin vaginal cream | Inserted into vagina 2 to 3 times per week |
| Estradiol | Estring | Inserted into the vagina once every 3 months |
|  | Vagifem tablet | Inserted into vagina twice a week |

in sexual activity. Although they may make intercourse more comfortable, vaginal moisturizers aren't a substitute for vaginal lubricants. However, you can use a lubricant as needed in addition to a moisturizer.

■ **Low-dose vaginal estrogen therapy.** For perimenopausal and postmenopausal women, reintroducing estrogen into the vaginal tissues on a regular basis can reverse vaginal dryness, thinning of the vaginal lining, and other age-related changes, as opposed to the temporary relief of dryness offered by lubricants and moisturizers. The following prescription-only products are available:

- **Vaginal creams.** Estrace, which contains 17-beta-estradiol, and Premarin, which contains conjugated estrogens, are vaginal creams that are inserted into the vagina two to three times per week. Note that estrogen cream should not be used as a lubricant before intercourse because it can be absorbed through a partner's skin.
- **Ring.** Estring is a low-dose vaginal ring containing 17-beta-estradiol that you insert into the vagina once every three months. It does not need to be removed before intercourse.
- **Tablet.** Vagifem is a tablet containing estradiol hemihydrate that is inserted into the vagina twice weekly using an applicator or your finger.

■ **Higher-dose estrogen therapy.** Estrogen products that increase levels of the hormone throughout the body, not just in the vagina, can ease menopausal symptoms such as hot flashes and night sweats—which, like vaginal dryness, can also interfere with a satisfying sex life. Because of research suggesting an increased risk of heart attack, stroke, blood clots, and breast cancer in women taking higher doses of estrogen, clinicians routinely advise women to use the lowest possible dose of estrogen for the shortest possible time to relieve their symptoms.

The following provides a brief over-

### Table 8: Hormone therapy for menopausal symptoms

These products increase blood levels of estrogen and treat both vaginal dryness and other menopausal symptoms such as hot flashes and night sweats. Women without a uterus can take estrogen by itself; those who have a uterus must take a progestin or progesterone in addition to estrogen (either separately or in a combination product) to minimize the risk of uterine cancer that can occur with estrogen alone. (Note: ß = beta)

| HORMONE(S) | TRADE NAME |
|---|---|
| **Oral estrogen (pills)** | |
| Conjugated equine estrogens | Premarin |
| Synthetic conjugated estrogens | Cenestin, Enjuvia |
| Esterified estrogens | Menest |
| 17ß-estradiol | Estrace, generics |
| Estrone (estropipate) | Ogen, Ortho-Est, generics |
| **Transdermal estrogen (patch, gel, cream, spray)** | |
| 17ß-estradiol patch | Alora, Climara, Esclim, Estraderm, Menostar, Vivelle-Dot, generics |
| 17ß-estradiol gel | Divigel, Elestrin, Estrogel |
| 17ß-estradiol cream | Estrasorb |
| 17ß-estradiol spray | Evamist |
| **Vaginal estrogen (ring)** | |
| Estradiol acetate | Femring |
| **Progestin pills** | |
| Medroxyprogesterone acetate | Provera, generics |
| Norethindrone | Micronor, Nor-QD, generics |
| Megestrol acetate | Megace |
| **Intrauterine progestin** | |
| Levonorgestrel IUS | Mirena |
| **Progesterone pill** | |
| Micronized progesterone USP | Prometrium |
| **Progesterone vaginal products** | |
| Progesterone gel | Crinone 8% |
| Progesterone vaginal tablet | Endometrin |
| **Combination estrogen-progestogen pills** | |
| Conjugated estrogens plus medroxyprogesterone acetate | Premphase, Prempro |
| Ethinyl estradiol plus norethindrone acetate | Femhrt |
| 17ß-estradiol plus norethindrone acetate | Activella |
| 17ß-estradiol plus norgestimate | Prefest |
| **Combination estrogen-progestogen patch** | |
| 17ß-estradiol plus norethindrone acetate | CombiPatch |
| 17ß-estradiol plus levonorgestrel | Climara Pro |

*Source: North American Menopause Society*

view of the different kinds of high-dose hormone preparations.

- **Pills.** These medications contain either estrogens, progestins, or both hormones together. Estrogen alone (called unopposed estrogen) is recommended only for women who have had a hysterectomy because taking the hormone by itself can raise the risk of developing uterine cancer. Adding a progestogen (a version of the hormone progesterone) to the formula protects against this risk. Examples of estrogen pills are Premarin, Cenestin, and Estrace. Oral progestogens include Provera, Micronor, and Prometrium. Combination pills include Premphase, Prempro, Femhrt, and Activella.

- **Patches.** Applied like a Band-Aid, patches deliver a continuous dose of estrogen for up to a week. Patches are worn on the abdomen or buttocks and are replaced every three to seven days. Typically, an oral progestogen is used along with the patch, although some patches contain both estrogen and progestogen. Because the estrogen enters the bloodstream without passing through the liver, it may be a more natural way to take estrogen. Some users report that the patch can itch or fall off. Examples of estrogen patches are Alora, Vivelle-Dot, Climara, and Menostar; combination patches that contain both estrogen and progestogen include CombiPatch and Climara Pro.

- **Gels, creams, and sprays.** In these therapies, hormones are applied to the skin. One product, EstroGel, comes in a clear, odorless, alcohol-based gel that's delivered from a metered-dose pump. The gel is applied once a day on one arm from the wrist to the shoulder. The gel dries completely in two to five minutes. Estrasorb is a cream that comes in individual foil packets and is rubbed into the thighs and buttocks. Evamist delivers estrogen through a metered-dose spray applied to a small area of the forearm.

- **Ring.** Femring is inserted into the vagina for three months. This higher-dose product treats hot flashes and vaginal dryness and should not be confused with the low-dose Estring, which treats only vaginal dryness.

### Sex therapy techniques

If your clinician feels your problem may benefit from nondrug therapy, he or she will recommend sex therapy. The sex therapist's role is to help you identify the thoughts, feelings, and behaviors that might be interfering with your sexual enjoyment. He or she will also encourage you to become more in touch with your erotic feelings and more comfortable with your body. In addition to sensate focus exercises, the therapist may encourage you to try a range of techniques, such as sexual fantasy training, masturbation exercises, and the use of erotica and vibrators. Because most women find that being able to share their feelings and wishes with their partner is a prerequisite for arousal, therapy will also concentrate on improving communication and enhancing feelings of intimacy between you and your partner.

## Vulvar and vaginal pain

A particularly distressing sexual problem for women is chronic vulvar or vaginal pain. About one in five American women may experience this problem at some point in her life. Like back pain or headache, pain in the vulva (vulvodynia) or vagina encompasses a variety of unpleasant sensations that may have psychological as well as physical causes. The pain can be diffuse and intermittent, it may appear when pressure is applied to certain areas, or it may emerge only when a woman is attempting sexual intercourse. A woman who experiences painful intercourse (dyspareunia) may become reluctant or unable to have sex, which can significantly strain an intimate relationship.

### Diagnosing the problem

Obstetricians and gynecologists report that pain during intercourse is a frequent complaint. If you have

---

#### A pill to boost desire?

An experimental drug called flibanserin, which was originally tested as an antidepressant, appears to boost female sexual desire. In several studies, premenopausal women who took flibanserin pills reported more sexually satisfying encounters and increased sexual desire compared with those who took a placebo. But the overall benefits were modest, and the drug's side effects include dizziness, fatigue, and nausea. An FDA advisory panel did not recommend approval of this drug, citing limited efficacy and potential side effects, although studies are ongoing.

## Coping with a history of sexual abuse

It's not surprising that people with a history of sexual abuse or rape are likely to develop sexual difficulties. While sexual abuse is more common in women, it also affects men.

Experts define childhood sexual abuse as occurring when a child engages in sexual activity for which she or he did not give consent, is unprepared for developmentally, or can't understand. It includes fondling and all forms of sexual contact with the child, even if the child is clothed. Abuse that doesn't involve touching, such as exhibitionism, voyeurism, or involving the child in pornography, is also included. Experts have stated that about 20% of girls and 9% of boys are involved in inappropriate sexual activities, but these figures are probably an underestimate because children often keep sexual abuse a secret.

Sexual assault or rape (any sexual act performed by one person on another without consent) is even more common: one in six women and one in 33 men report having experienced an attempted or completed rape at some time in their lives. But in both sexes, reported rapes are probably only a fraction of those actually committed.

As you might expect, these experiences often affect a person's attitudes and feelings about sex. For instance, chronic pelvic pain—an obvious barrier to satisfying sex—is more likely in women with a history of sexual abuse. What may be surprising, yet not uncommon, is when a person suddenly develops sexual difficulties after previously appearing to enjoy a good sexual relationship with his or her partner. In some cases, problems crop up after the relationship undergoes a major change. After a couple makes a formal commitment to each other, for example, a woman with a history of sexual abuse may now feel that she is part of a family, with its concomitant obligations and expectations. If a family member abused her, she may now recall those experiences and be reluctant to have sex. Likewise, the birth of a child may trigger memories of childhood abuse. Or the memory may reappear when the child reaches the age the person was when the abuse occurred.

For couples facing such problems, a treatment plan might include such steps as these:

- individual and group therapy for the survivor of abuse
- simultaneous individual or group therapy for the partner
- couples or sex therapy to educate the couple about the sexual impact of abuse and to help them find ways to stay close and connected
- couples or sex therapy to address any sexual or complicated relationship issues once the survivor of abuse feels ready to do so.

---

this problem, your clinician will ask you about your symptoms. For example, he or she will ask you to describe the type of pain (burning, shooting, sharp, or dull) and to identify its location (deep within your vagina or around the vaginal opening). You may also be asked to point out the sensitive areas using a handheld mirror.

Next, you'll have a complete physical exam. For women with vaginal pain, a pelvic exam can be uncomfortable. A good clinician will understand your concerns and take extra care to perform the exam slowly and gently. When inserting a speculum or several gloved fingers, he or she will assess whether involuntary vaginal tightening (vaginismus) occurs.

One important element of the diagnostic workup for vulvar pain is the Q-tip test. Using a moistened cotton swab, your clinician will gently touch several sites on the inner labia and around the vaginal opening. You'll be asked to report the intensity of the pain on a scale of 1 to 10. Pain in certain areas during the test may indicate an inflammatory condition known as vulvar vestibulitis.

Your clinician will also look for signs of age-related vaginal changes that can make intercourse uncomfortable. Finally, you may be tested to rule out the presence of an infection.

### Types of pain

Vulvar and vaginal pain is categorized based on your symptoms and what the clinician finds during your evaluation. These are some of the more common conditions.

■ **Vaginal atrophy.** Lower estrogen levels cause the vaginal lining to thin and secretions to diminish. The vagina also becomes shorter and less elastic, and the vaginal opening narrows. The result is often dryness and irritation, which can make intercourse or pelvic examinations painful or impossible. Thinning of the vaginal lining combined with changes in the pH balance can make the vagina vulnerable to infection—a condition known as atrophic vaginitis. Urinary tract infections are more common as well, as the urethra also has estrogen receptors. If untreated, atrophy may lead to further thinning and ulceration of the vagina.

■ **Vaginismus.** This condition is characterized by involuntary spasms of the muscles in the outer third of the vagina in response to any attempt at entry. It makes intercourse difficult or impossible. Vaginismus can be the result of past sexual abuse, lack of sexual experience, or fear of or aversion to sexual activity. It may also develop as a secondary effect of other pain-related conditions, such as vaginal atrophy.

■ **Vulvodynia.** Vulvodynia is pain with no identifiable cause that may come and go in different areas, including the clitoris, perineum, mons pubis, and inner thighs. Symptoms include burning, stinging, and irritation. The condition can make sexual intercourse uncomfortable or impossible.

■ **Vulvar vestibulitis.** This is a condition in which the inner labia and vaginal opening become chronically inflamed and irritated. Pressure to the area from any source—such as the entry of a penis, insertion of a tampon, contact with a bicycle seat, or even wearing tight pants—can cause extreme tenderness. The exact cause of vulvar vestibulitis is unknown.

■ **Pelvic pain.** Pelvic pain refers to pain inside your pelvis. There are many possible causes, including adhesions, interstitial cystitis, and endometriosis. Adhesions are bands of tissue that form in response to injury or infection. Scars from an episiotomy (an incision in the area between the vagina and anus to enlarge the vagina during childbirth) can create adhesions; so can abdominal surgery, including C-sections and hysterectomies. In some cases, adhesions bind internal organs together or to the pelvic wall. Interstitial cystitis, which is inflammation within the bladder, is another cause of pelvic pain. So is endometriosis, which causes tissue from the uterus to grow outside of its normal location. All of these conditions can cause painful sex and may inhibit a woman's ability to have an orgasm.

**Treating vaginal pain**

Treatment of vaginal pain depends on the root of the problem. Vaginal atrophy can be treated with nonhormonal lubricants or moisturizers that allow a return to sexual activity or estrogen treatments that can reverse the atrophy. If vaginismus is a reaction to pain, sex therapy in combination with physical therapy can alleviate the problem once the pain has been treated. Since vulvodynia and vulvar vestibulitis have no known cause or cure, treatment usually centers around pain management techniques. Sex therapy can also help a woman deal with the effect of the pain on her sexuality and rebuild a pleasurable sex life.

■ **Medication.** An assortment of medications are used for vaginal pain, with varying degrees of success. Steroid creams are effective in treating vaginal inflammation. If the primary cause of the pain is vaginal atrophy (thinning and dryness), low doses of estrogen applied directly to the vagina—in the form of a cream, tablet, or ring—can help restore natural lubrication (see "Low-dose vaginal estrogen therapy," page 33). If the pain stems from an infection, your health care provider may prescribe antibiotic creams or pills. Anesthetic ointments are sometimes used. In the case of vulvar vestibulitis, interferon injections have been successful in controlling the inflammation. Other medications such as tricyclic antidepressants and gabapentin (approved to treat seizures and certain pain syndromes) work in some cases.

> **Tips for making sex more comfortable**
>
> If sex is uncomfortable, here are some things you can do to reduce your discomfort and enhance your pleasure.
>
> - Relax and practice Kegel exercises to make sure you aren't tightening up.
> - Use plenty of lubricant with both sexual stimulation and intercourse and consider regular use of long-acting vaginal moisturizers.
> - If you are postmenopausal, consider using low-dose vaginal estrogen therapy.
> - Use a topical anesthetic gel with a 5% concentration of the local anesthetic lidocaine to ease burning during intercourse. You can get this with a prescription from your health care provider.
> - Use lubricated, graduated vaginal dilators (see page 38) regularly, if your vagina tightens involuntarily when intercourse is attempted (vaginismus), or if your vagina feels like it has become short or narrow over time.
> - Apply a frozen gel-pack wrapped in a towel to your vulva to ease irritation after manual sexual stimulation or intercourse.
> - After intercourse, urinate (to avoid an infection) and rinse your vulva in cool water.
>
> Adapted from "Self-Help Tips for Vulvar Skin Care," with permission from the National Vulvodynia Association, www.nva.org.

## Alternative therapies for sexual problems

Can an herb or supplement improve your sex life? The market is flooded with herbal products whose manufacturers claim they can, but consumers should treat these claims with skepticism. Remember, in every study of a medication for sexual dysfunction, placebo patches, gels, and pills are very effective!

Most of the creams and herbal supplements available over the counter and sold on the Internet have not been studied rigorously. Since the FDA doesn't regulate the use and dosage of herbal products, their safety and effectiveness are unknown. Dosages can vary widely from product to product and even pill to pill. Keep in mind, too, that "natural" doesn't mean harmless. Herbal products can cause side effects and interact with other medications.

Also, what's listed on the label is not necessarily what's inside the bottle. This is illustrated by a 2006 FDA warning that urged consumers to avoid a variety of dietary supplements that claim to treat erectile dysfunction and improve sexual performance. The FDA found that some products contained sildenafil, vardenafil, or substances that are nearly identical to these medications. But none of these chemicals were listed on the products' labels. In fact, the packaging was misleading. According to the FDA, the packaging claimed that the products were "all natural" and did not contain the active ingredients used in FDA-approved erectile dysfunction drugs.

This poses a serious health risk to consumers who might take such a product unaware that it could interact with other medications. Chemicals such as sildenafil or vardenafil can interact with nitrates (which are commonly used to treat angina and heart failure) and cause blood pressure to drop to dangerously low levels.

There is a dizzying array of other products marketed for improving sexual function. The chart below examines a handful of commonly known alternative therapies. But medical experts agree that if you choose to use pills, it's best to opt for well-tested, FDA-approved medications. If you do decide to use an alternative therapy, tell your clinician about it so he or she can watch for possible side effects and drug interactions.

### Common alternative therapies

| NAME | WHAT IS IT? | HOW DOES IT WORK? | IS IT SAFE? |
|---|---|---|---|
| Yohimbine (Yocon) | Oral treatment for erectile dysfunction. Derived from the bark of a West African evergreen. | Opens blood vessels in the skin and mucous membranes. May be helpful for men who can't take Viagra, Cialis, or Levitra, although its effectiveness has not been clearly established. | Side effects include anxiety, insomnia, increased heart rate and blood pressure, tremors, nervousness, irritability, and dizziness. |
| Ginkgo biloba | Chinese herb said to improve libido and erectile function. Available in pill form. | Opens blood vessels and increases blood flow. May be helpful if your erectile problems are the result of inadequate blood flow. | Can cause headache, stomach upset, dizziness, diarrhea, and skin reaction. Has a blood-thinning effect, so should not be used with anticoagulant medications or before surgery. |
| Dehydro-epiand-rosterone (DHEA) | A naturally occurring hormone that is converted into testosterone and estrogen in the body. Said to improve libido, female arousal and orgasm, and erectile dysfunction. | Increases the body's testosterone and estrogen levels. May improve libido and erectile function in isolated cases, but little reliable evidence on its effectiveness exists. More information is also needed on long-term effects. | May cause growth of facial hair and acne in women. High doses could cause liver problems and lower "good" cholesterol. The long-term risks of male hormones in women are not known, but may include heart disease and breast cancer. |
| Avlimil | A dietary supplement that contains 11 herbs, including some (black cohosh, licorice, red raspberry, red clover, and kudzu) that have estrogenic effects; said to improve female sexual dysfunction. | Advertised as relieving menopause symptoms and "restoring well-being," in addition to enhancing female sexual functions. | Research suggests it works no better than a placebo, and one study in mice suggested that Avlimil may stimulate the growth of certain types of breast cancer. |
| Zestra | A plant-based arousal oil for women made from a blend of borage seed oil, evening primrose oil, vitamin E, and other herbs. This topical treatment is applied to the clitoris and labia during foreplay. Shown in a small clinical study to help enhance sexual function in women with sexual arousal disorder. | The makers of the oil claim that it increases genital blood flow and improves the workings of the genital sensory nerves. Contains large amounts of a fatty acid that the body converts to prostaglandin, which helps increase blood flow and nerve conduction. | When used as directed, few side effects have been reported thus far, except for possible mild skin irritation. |

- **Vaginal dilators.** These products consist of a set of plastic round-tipped cylinders that range in size from small (with a diameter of about ¾ inch) to large (the diameter of a fully erect penis). Regular use of dilators, for about five minutes every night, can dramatically increase comfort with intercourse for many women. Trained physical therapists can explain the technique, but a woman can do the exercises at home at her own pace. There are many different techniques, but typically, a woman starts by inserting a small dilator into her vagina, leaving it in place for about one minute, removing it, and then reinserting it. This exercise should be repeated about five times over five minutes nightly. Dilators always should be well-lubricated and comfortable. Over time, a woman uses successively larger dilators until the exercises are comfortable with a dilator the size of a fully erect penis. The process effectively enables the woman to stretch the vagina and also stop involuntary tightening of the vaginal opening (vaginismus).

- **Pelvic floor physical therapy.** This technique is very effective for many women in treating unremitting vaginal or pelvic pain. It uses hands-on physical therapy to relax muscles in the lower pelvis. The physical therapist uses a massage-like technique, known as myofascial release, to help stretch and release the fascia (connective tissue between the skin and underlying muscle and bones). Pelvic floor physical therapy is also used to treat other causes of dyspareunia, such as vulvodynia and vulvar vestibulitis, as well as urinary incontinence.

- **Behavior management.** Biofeedback has been used successfully to control vulvar pain. You begin by inserting special sensors into the vagina or rectum to help identify overly tense pelvic floor muscles, which can be a cause of vulvar pain. Then, you perform targeted exercises to relax these muscles. A physical therapist with expertise in the muscles of the pelvic floor will help you with biofeedback. Acupuncture or the use of cold packs may also be helpful.

- **Sex therapy.** Painful intercourse usually causes people to feel anxious about sexual activity and as a result, they often avoid it completely. Eventually this fear and withdrawal become as formidable as the pain itself. The fear of pain can also contribute to performance anxiety, creating a vicious cycle. By working with a sex therapist, you and your partner can learn to focus on sexual and sensual activities that are pleasurable and not at all painful. The therapist will use structured activities such as sensate focus techniques to direct your attention to activities and parts of the body that don't provoke anxiety or cause pain. You can then begin specific treatments to promote comfortable intercourse, such as regular use of vaginal dilators or pelvic floor physical therapy.

# Orgasm difficulties

Few aspects of human sexuality have incurred the intense debate that has surrounded orgasm. As scientists struggle to quantify this holy grail of sexual experience, certain questions come up repeatedly: are orgasms the same for women and men? Is an orgasm primarily a psychological or physiological experience? Do women have more than one kind of orgasm, and if so, which type is "better"? The speculation on these points will no doubt continue, but the highly individual and subjective nature of orgasms forces another important question: when does an orgasm difficulty become a dysfunction? As with other sexual problems, an orgasm that is premature, delayed, or absent warrants special attention only when it causes you or your partner distress.

### Problems in men

The amount of penile and other stimulation a man needs before ejaculating varies greatly. A young man who is highly aroused may feel the urge to ejaculate very quickly after entering his partner. With experience, most men learn to anticipate the moment of ejaculation and employ techniques to slow their orgasm.

As a man ages, several changes take place. An older man ejaculates less semen, so the fluid may release less forcefully. Having less ejaculate translates into less intense pressure for release. This allows a mature man to enjoy a longer period of stimulation before feeling an overwhelming urge to ejaculate.

Often, men can adjust lovemaking routines to accommodate natural age-related occurrences. However, some of the following conditions can disrupt a man's sexual pleasure and that of his partner.

■ **Premature ejaculation.** Premature ejaculation is a common problem in which a man ejaculates as soon as or shortly after intercourse starts or even before he enters his partner. It often leads to anxiety that this will occur again. The woman may become frustrated as she finds her sexual arousal continually thwarted, and as a result she may lose interest in sex.

Rarely, early ejaculation can be traced to a medical problem. Your clinician will want to rule out urologic conditions, diseases, or an injury to the nervous system.

If an underlying physical problem isn't to blame, treatment usually involves medication, sex therapy, or both. Ironically, an adverse side effect of certain antidepressants can be put to positive use in treating premature ejaculation. In several studies of paroxetine (Paxil), sertraline (Zoloft), and clomipramine (Anafranil), men reported having more time before ejaculation and greater sexual satisfaction for themselves and their partners.

In sex therapy, the therapist will help you and your partner explore and address the issues that may be contributing to the dysfunction. In addition, you'll learn behavioral exercises such as sensate focus and a start-stop technique that is often very helpful. You'll also be encouraged to adapt your foreplay and lovemaking style to increase your sexual enjoyment.

■ **Delayed ejaculation or orgasm.** Delayed ejaculation occurs when a man is able to have an erection but isn't able to ejaculate. There's no "right" amount of time for a man to take to reach orgasm. An older man will generally need more prolonged stimulation for arousal and orgasm. Also, some men reach orgasm much more easily through manual and oral stimulation. Because the urge to ejaculate lessens with age, an older man may be able to enjoy intercourse without needing to ejaculate every time. However, if the urge is present but orgasm fails to occur after a lengthy period of intercourse, he may give up trying. Alternately, the man's female partner may need to halt lovemaking because of vaginal discomfort. Delayed ejaculation is a relatively rare problem, affecting only 3% to 8% of men.

When assessing the problem, one of the first things your health care provider will do is ask you which medications you take. Many antidepressants,

### ▶ Embrace yoga to enhance your sex life

Rooted in Indian philosophy, yoga is an ancient method of relaxation, exercise, and healing that's gained a wide following in the United States. Research suggests that yoga can ease anxiety, arthritis, and a host of other mental and physical woes. Yoga—from the Sanskrit word meaning "union"—may even enhance women's sexual function, according to a 2009 study in *The Journal of Sexual Medicine*.

The study involved 40 sexually active women, ages 22 to 55, who were enrolled in a yoga camp in India. Each filled out a standard sexual function questionnaire at the beginning and the end of the 12-week camp, which entailed an hour of yoga practice each day followed by breathing and relaxation. Researchers found that the women's sexual function scores in all six domains (desire, arousal, lubrication, orgasm, satisfaction, and pain) had improved by the end of the camp—especially among women who were over age 45. And nearly three-quarters of the women said their sex lives improved following the yoga camp.

If you'd like to try yoga, classes and instructional DVDs abound. By some estimates, 75% of all American gyms now offer yoga classes. Many different styles are available, and although many forms of yoga are safe, some are strenuous and may not be appropriate for everyone. In particular, elderly people or those with mobility problems may want to check first with a clinician before trying yoga.

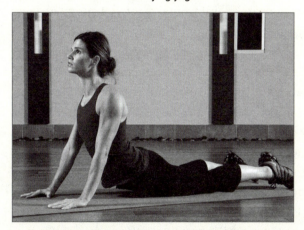

This pose, known as snake or cobra pose, is one of the asanas (yoga postures) done by the women in the study. Researchers specifically chose asanas believed to affect factors such as mood, joint movements, and muscles in the abdomen and pelvis for the study.

blood pressure medications, and medications for obsessive-compulsive disorder can produce orgasm difficulties. To correct the problem, your clinician may recommend reducing the dosage of the drug, changing the frequency at which you take it, or switching to a different drug altogether. Don't stop taking a medication or alter your dose without speaking first to your health care provider. Another possibility is to take bupropion, which may counteract the sexual side effects of other medications.

The inability of a man to come to orgasm through penetration or in the presence of his partner may have a learned behavioral or psychological origin. A sex therapist can explore how you have learned to have orgasm on your own. You may be encouraged to work on bridging—in other words, beginning with the method you typically use and gradually including ways that will involve your partner.

The therapist will also explore and then address the possible behavioral and emotional issues at the core of your inability to have an orgasm. He or she can guide you in the use of devices or masturbation techniques to help you overcome the problem. However, the primary goal will always be to help you fully experience pleasure during all kinds of sexual play, with or without reaching orgasm.

**Problems in women**

A common complaint from women is a complete lack of orgasms or an inability to have an orgasm with a partner (especially during intercourse). In a survey of 862 sexually active older women, about 13% of the women reported that they had experienced orgasms rarely or not at all during the past six months. As with other sexual dysfunctions, female orgasm difficulties can stem from physical and emotional causes, as well as issues involving the couple's relationship or sexual practices. Often, it's the result of a combination of factors. Remember, however, that women can also enjoy sex without reaching orgasm. Lack of orgasm is only a problem if it's bothering you.

Your clinician will investigate possible physical causes. These might include vaginal atrophy, nerve damage from pelvic surgery (such as a hysterectomy) or even long-distance bicycle riding, vaginal pain, depression, or side effects of medications such as antidepressants.

Regardless of the findings, sex therapy is very effective. The therapist will first ask whether you've ever been able to have an orgasm—either through masturbation or with a partner.

If you've never had an orgasm, the therapist will explore issues in your past such as sexual abuse or negative messages and attitudes about sex or masturbation. The therapist will also encourage you to become more familiar with your body and what pleases you sexually. Books and videos are often helpful; the therapist may suggest that you buy a vibrator and experiment with using it to stimulate yourself, eventually in front of your partner if you're comfortable doing so. This technique is often successful in helping a woman learn to have orgasms. The orgasm rate is somewhat lower when these women have intercourse with their partners, but most report that after therapy, they enjoy sex more and have a more relaxed attitude about it.

In some cases, women enter sex therapy with the ability to have orgasms through masturbation, but not with a partner. The therapist will approach this situation by exploring how the partners stimulate each other. He or she will also delve into emotional issues that may be getting in the way, such as how you and your partner relate to each other and what your orgasms mean to both of you. Another important element of treatment is sensate focus exercises. If difficulty communicating your sexual needs is at the root of the problem, these exercises can help the two of you develop these skills. By placing the emphasis on enjoyment rather than reaching orgasm, a woman can relax and focus on her own pleasure.

Sex therapy underscores that orgasmic responses vary. At one extreme are the rare reports of women having orgasms from fantasy alone or just from having their breasts caressed. Somewhere in the middle are women who can, in one position or another, reach orgasm during intercourse. However, still other women find they need direct clitoral stimulation. A good therapist will reassure couples that there is no one right way to experience sexual pleasure and encourage them to adapt their lovemaking style to best suit their needs.

**SPECIAL SECTION**

# Everything you always wanted to know about sex therapy

Sexual problems are nearly always intertwined with psychological and relationship issues. As a result, treating the physical problem (if one is present) is only half the job. If sexual issues persist for any length of time, performance anxiety, anger, frustration, low self-esteem, lack of physical affection between you and your partner, and a sense of hopelessness can further harm your sex life. So can a tendency to blame yourself or your partner for the problem. Most people need help repairing the emotional distance created by the problem before they can regain a healthy sexual relationship.

Licensed sex therapists are particularly well suited to this task. Although they're qualified to understand the same broad emotional issues as individual or couples therapists, sex therapists have advanced training in addressing specific sexual problems, and they use a more targeted approach. Initially, underlying personal dilemmas and relationship conflicts are addressed mainly in the context of your sexual problems. As a result, sex therapy will probably return you to sexual functioning sooner than traditional counseling. However, as the sexual issue is being resolved, many people choose to continue working with the sex therapist to tackle deeper personal and relationship issues.

### What to expect during sex therapy

To understand what takes place during a sex therapy session, it's important to know what doesn't happen. Contrary to what some people may think, you will not be physically intimate with each other while the therapist is watching. If having to discuss your sex life is an obstacle to getting help, you can rest assured that the sex therapist will not push you too quickly. Also, remember than an essential part of the treatment is learning how to talk about your sexual feelings more comfortably.

The role of sex therapy is to help people explore the nature and possible causes of their sexual concerns, better communicate their sexual needs and preferences, and expand their repertoire of sensual and sexual activities. By increasing the overall pleasure and intimacy of sexual contact, a couple will be able to enjoy expressions of sensuality that are free from what are often the goal-driven pressures of intercourse and orgasm.

William H. Masters and Virginia E. Johnson pioneered sex therapy in the 1960s. The original model consisted of an intensive two-week treatment program revolving around daily therapy sessions. Couples traveled to the Masters and Johnson Institute and stayed in a hotel for the duration of the treatment. Although intensive weeklong or weekend programs are still available at a few centers around the country, most sex therapists use a modified format in which the couple meets with the therapist in his or her office for weekly 50-minute sessions. There are certified sex therapists in most major cities, so you most likely won't need to travel far from home to get help.

Much of the behavioral and relationship-building work of sex therapy is actually done at home between meetings with the therapist. After the comprehensive assessment is complete and the couple feels comfortable with and trusts the therapist, the therapist will probably assign behavioral exercises to practice at home. You'll be asked to focus on your feelings, sensations, and thoughts during the home assignment and to discuss them with the therapist in the next session.

The therapist may also serve as a sex educator. In many cases—for example, with age-related changes or vaginal pain syndromes—understanding the physiological basis of the problem often goes a long way toward relieving your anxiety, as well as your partner's. The therapist will discuss such issues with you during therapy sessions and may suggest useful books and DVDs. He or she will also help you question erroneous beliefs and assumptions that stand in the way of enjoyable sex, such as "All sexual contact must lead to intercourse," "The man must be in charge of the sexual activity," or "Foreplay is only for teenagers and isn't really sex."

Sex therapy can also help you learn to take some control of other factors that inhibit your sexual enjoyment. By understanding where stressors lie and how they influence sexual functioning, a couple can take steps to create a relaxed, distraction-free environment for sex. Older couples, who often need more time and stimulation to feel aroused and reach orgasm, may find they benefit from making an extra effort to set a leisurely romantic mood.

### Sensate focus: The foundation of sex therapy

The cornerstone of sex therapy is a series of behavioral exercises called sensate focus exercises. These highly structured touching activities are designed to help you overcome performance anxiety and increase your comfort with physical intimacy. Sensate focus training also helps teach you about your partner's body as well as your own.

Initially, the couple agrees to refrain from intercourse or genital stimulation until the later stages of treatment. This helps dispel anxiety that's built up around sexual performance and allows you to establish new patterns of relating sensually, sexually, and emotionally. Couples and therapists also discuss how frequently the couple will perform the assigned exercises between therapy sessions.

### Sex therapy in the age of erectile dysfunction drugs

When Viagra was first introduced, some sex therapists worried they would shortly be out of a job. But they soon learned otherwise.

Erectile dysfunction can set in motion a cycle of emotional and relationship problems that need addressing. Likewise, an instant "cure" in the form of a pill can uncover other sources of sexual dysfunction, such a low libido, difficulties with arousal, or vaginal pain from menopausal changes. If Viagra, Levitra, or Cialis allows you to resume sex after a hiatus, a sex therapist can help you transition back to sexual activity. These are some of the sex therapist's tasks:

- Determining whether both members of the couple are comfortable with and committed to using the drug.

- Discussing the conditions each person needs for pleasurable sex. For the woman, this may mean more romantic time that includes talking, affection, and sensual touching before moving to sexual activity. The therapist will also encourage the couple to learn how to adjust their lovemaking to incorporate the waiting period (if there is one) while the medication takes effect. (This interval may actually serve to encourage the type of sensual lovemaking that sex therapists recommend.)

- Exploring expectations for resuming sex. The therapist can help you accept that sex will sometimes be just okay, that arousal problems may still occur, and that these medications won't work without desire and physical stimulation.

- Addressing other sexual issues the man may have, such as ejaculatory problems.

- Delving into emotional and relationship issues that are interfering with intimacy.

- Devising strategies to deal with instances of unsuccessful intercourse.

Occasionally, couples are reluctant to complete the homework assignments. This too can be revealing. By delving into the roots of this resistance, the therapist can better understand the origins of the problem.

### How it works

Sensate focus techniques progress through several stages. The therapist will provide a detailed individualized scenario for the couple to follow at each level, but here is an overview.

- **Sensate focus I.** To start off, you're encouraged to spend about a half-hour per person caressing each other's naked bodies front and back, from head to toe, but avoiding the breasts and the genitals. You and your partner take turns being the

---

### A sample scenario: Treating a woman with low desire

To give you a better sense of how sex therapists work with couples, Suki Hanfling, one of the medical editors of this report, discusses how she might approach an issue she often deals with in her practice: a 60-something married woman with low desire.

It's not unusual for a woman to call and ask if she can come in to discuss her issue alone, without her partner, because she feels that it's "her" problem. In that situation, I would explore her feelings about sex therapy and her reasons for that preference. I might then explain that even if she doesn't believe her partner is part of the problem, he is definitely part of the solution.

Sometimes the husband is reluctant to participate. I usually encourage the woman to invite her husband to come to at least one session by explaining that it would help me to understand his point of view and feelings about their sexual relationship.

I begin by creating a safe and comfortable environment so that each person can describe in detail how he or she views the problem—how and when it started, any ideas about possible contributing factors, and what they as a couple have tried so far to remedy it.

When the problem of low desire develops later in life, I explain that health and hormonal changes after age 50 often translate to less spontaneous and less compelling desire than people usually feel when they are younger. I also explain how for some women, sexual desire can follow sexual arousal, especially if there is no pressure to have sex.

I also explore the history of the couple's courtship and overall relationship. I usually ask how many hours they spend each week just enjoying each other's company. If they report that they hardly spend any time alone together, I recommend that we begin by focusing on their relationship and then address their sexual concerns. I encourage them to identify the strengths of their earlier relationship (sexual and otherwise) and suggest that if they are willing to work together, they can build on those strengths.

Women with low desire often come to therapy because of their partner's concern about the lack of sex. I ask whether either of them ever misses the physical affection and closeness that comes with sex. If the answer is yes, we explore how they might be more physically affectionate without feeling pressure to have sex. We also talk about how each person initiates or turns down a request for sex, and how they might communicate their feelings in a less pressuring or negative way. I also encourage the woman to share what she hopes her husband will do for her—both sexually and emotionally—and vice versa.

Early in the process, I usually meet individually with each person to get a more detailed understanding of their sexual concerns and history that they might not have been comfortable sharing with each other. We discuss whether they have had similar difficulties in any prior relationships and whether there are concerns about any other aspects of their current sexual life. Then I suggest things they can do at home. For example, I may recommend books, DVDs, or a sensate focus exercise. Although sensate focus is unlikely to increase desire, it can often illuminate some of the contributing issues.

For a woman with low desire, I might suggest she write about her ideal sexual encounter and see what she discovers. It's up to her if she wants to share it. She could also practice some form of relaxation, read erotica, or take a daily fantasy break for a few minutes, during which she recalls a pleasant sexual experience from her past or an erotic encounter from a book or movie. If she is unable to conjure up a sexual fantasy, I encourage her to periodically stop during the day and pay attention to what she is feeling both emotionally and physically.

As therapy progresses and couples begin to be sexual together, other problems sometimes arise. If either person feels concerned about how quickly he or she becomes aroused, I share an old saying: when it comes to sex, men are like microwaves and women are like crock-pots, because it takes women longer to warm up. But the truth is that as men age, they often become more like crock-pots! In that spirit, I recommend that couples think of the warm-up period, kissing, sensate focus, or foreplay as all being part of lovemaking. I encourage them to expand their definition of sex to include sensuality, intimacy, passion, and playfulness, which can help take the focus off performance and encourage them to be more mindful and in the moment.

**SPECIAL SECTION** | **Everything you always wanted to know about sex therapy**

## Overcoming anxiety about sex therapy

If you think sex therapy may be helpful but you're still uneasy about it, there are several ways to learn more about this treatment. Sexual self-help books and DVDs often describe exercises that a sex therapist might assign. Your primary care provider, gynecologist, or urologist may also be able to tell you something about the process.

Even if they understand what's involved in sex therapy, couples may be hesitant to take the first step. Anxieties may revolve around the fear that something serious is wrong with them, that sex therapy will hurt their relationship by focusing too much on the problem, or that if the therapy doesn't work it means the situation is hopeless. During an initial phone call, a sex therapist will be able to address these issues and very likely ease your anxiety.

Sex therapy is most successful when both partners are willing participants. However, if one partner is resistant, the other may seek treatment alone. In this case, the sex therapist may encourage the hesitant partner to attend for at least one session in order to discuss his or her thoughts on the issue. If the partner is unwilling to engage in therapy even to this extent, it's still possible for the other partner to benefit from the process.

---

giver and receiver of pleasure so you can concentrate fully on each sensation and your reaction to it. However, if this creates too much anxiety or is too intimate for the couple, the therapist may recommend beginning simply by holding hands or giving each other back rubs. During these initial exercises, the emphasis is on the giver touching in a way he or she enjoys (and that is pleasurable to the receiver as well).

### Finding a sex therapist

There are several approaches you can take to finding a qualified sex therapist. Your general health care provider, gynecologist, or urologist may be able to make a referral. Also, if you're working with an individual or couples therapist, he or she may direct you to a sex therapist. Another good source is the American Association of Sexuality Educators, Counselors, and Therapists, an organization that certifies sex therapists (see "Resources," page 48).

Once you have a name, take the following steps to determine whether the person is a good match for you:

- Call the sex therapist. Some therapists will talk with you on the phone for 15 or 20 minutes to describe their philosophy and approach to treatment and address any questions or concerns you may have.

- Ask about the approach used, the frequency of sessions, the possible duration of therapy, and the fees involved. Some insurance plans cover some or even all the cost of sex therapy, just as they do couples therapy or other counseling. However, you need to have an approved diagnosis to justify receiving compensation.

- Be sure that the therapist has extensive training and experience in both couples therapy and working directly with sexual problems.

- Schedule a first visit. Having an initial meeting is not a commitment to ongoing therapy. Use the session to get to know the therapist and gauge whether you feel comfortable and think you and your partner can benefit from working with him or her. If at all possible, both you and your partner should attend this meeting.

■ **Sensate focus II.** These exercises incorporate the lessons from sensate focus I, but the focus expands to the kind of touch the receiver wants. He or she takes an active role in explaining or showing his or her partner what kind of touch is enjoyable. Partners still take turns being the giver and receiver during each session.

■ **Sensate focus III.** Building on the previous sessions, these exercises expand to include touching the breasts and genitals, but not exclusively. The couple is encouraged to continue focusing on the sensations involved and on communicating what they enjoy and want sexually, rather than the goal of orgasm.

■ **Sensate focus IV.** At this point, the couple is allowed to enjoy mutual touching and stimulation to the point of orgasm. If all goes well, the couple can proceed to intercourse.

Depending on the needs of the couple, the sex therapist typically uses other behavioral techniques and treatment strategies. ▼

# Helping yourself to a better sex life

Whether the problem is big or small, there are many things you can do to get your sex life back on track. Communicating with your partner, maintaining a healthy lifestyle, availing yourself of some of the many excellent self-help materials on the market, and just having fun can help you weather tough times.

## Talking to your partner

Many couples find it difficult to talk about sex even under the best of circumstances. When sexual problems occur, feelings of hurt, shame, guilt, and resentment can halt conversation altogether. Because good communication is a cornerstone of a healthy relationship, establishing a dialogue is the first step not only to a better sex life, but also to a closer emotional bond. Here are some tips for tackling this sensitive subject.

■ **Find the right time to talk.** There are two types of sexual conversations: the ones you have in the bedroom and the ones you have elsewhere. It's perfectly appropriate to tell your partner what feels good in the middle of lovemaking, but it's best to wait until you're in a more neutral setting to discuss larger issues, such as mismatched sexual desire or orgasm troubles.

■ **Avoid criticizing.** Couch suggestions in positive terms, such as, "I really love it when you touch my hair lightly that way," rather than focusing on the negatives. Approach a sexual issue as a problem to be solved together rather than an exercise in assigning blame.

■ **Confide in your partner about changes in your body.** If hot flashes are keeping you up at night or menopause has made your vagina dry, talk to your partner about these things. It's much better that he know what's really going on rather than interpret these physical changes as lack of interest. Likewise, if you're a man and you no longer get an erection just from the thought of sex, show your partner how to stimulate you rather than let her believe she isn't attractive enough to arouse you anymore.

■ **Be honest.** You may think you're protecting your partner's feelings by faking an orgasm, but in reality you're starting down a slippery slope. As challenging as it is to talk about any sexual problem, the difficulty level skyrockets once the issue is buried under years of lies, hurt, and resentment.

■ **Don't equate love with sexual performance.** Create an atmosphere of caring and tenderness; touch and kiss often. Don't blame yourself or your partner for your sexual difficulties. Focus instead on maintaining emotional and physical intimacy in your relationship.

For older couples, another potentially sensitive subject that's worth discussing is what will happen after one partner dies. In couples who enjoy a healthy sex life, the surviving partner will likely want to seek out a new partner. Expressing your openness to that possibility while you are both still alive will likely relieve guilt and make the process less difficult for the surviving partner later.

## Using self-help strategies

Treating sexual problems is easier now than ever before. Revolutionary medications and professional sex therapists are there if you need them. But you may be able to resolve minor sexual issues by making a few adjustments in your lovemaking style. Here are some things you can try at home.

■ **Educate yourself.** Plenty of good self-help materials are available for every type of sexual issue. Browse the Internet (but see "Sex in the Internet age," page 47) or your local bookstore, pick out a few resources that apply to you, and use them to help you and your partner become better informed about the problem. If talking directly is too difficult, you and your partner can underline passages that you particularly like and show them to each other.

■ **Give yourself time.** As you age, your sexual responses slow down. You and your partner can improve your chances of success by finding a quiet, comfortable, interruption-free setting for sex. Also, understand that the physical changes in your body mean that you'll need more time to get aroused and reach orgasm. When you think about it, spending more time having sex isn't a bad thing; working these physical necessities into your lovemaking routine can open up doors to a new kind of sexual experience.

■ **Use lubrication.** Often, the vaginal dryness that begins in perimenopause can be easily corrected with lubricating liquids and gels. Use these freely to avoid painful sex—a problem that can snowball into flagging libido and growing relationship tensions. Regular use of long-acting vaginal moisturizers or low-dose vaginal estrogen therapy are other effective options.

■ **Maintain physical affection.** Even if you're tired, tense, or upset about the problem, engaging in kissing and cuddling is essential for maintaining an emotional and physical bond.

■ **Practice touching.** The sensate focus techniques that sex therapists use can help you re-establish physical intimacy without feeling pressured. Many self-help books and educational videos offer variations on these exercises. You may also want to ask your partner to touch you in a manner that he or she would like to be touched. This will give you a better sense of how much pressure, from gentle to firm, you should use.

■ **Try different positions.** Developing a repertoire of different sexual positions not only adds interest to lovemaking, but can also help overcome problems. For example, the increased stimulation to the G-spot that occurs when a man enters his partner from behind can help some women reach orgasm.

■ **Write down your fantasies.** This exercise can help you explore possible activities you think might be a turn-on for you or your partner. Try thinking of an experience or a movie that aroused you and then share your memory with your partner. This is especially helpful for people with low desire.

■ **Do Kegel exercises.** Both men and women can improve their sexual fitness by exercising their pelvic floor muscles. To do these exercises, tighten the muscle you would use if you were trying to stop urine in midstream. Hold the contraction for two or three seconds, then release. Repeat 10 times. Try to do five sets a day. These exercises can be done anywhere—while driving, sitting at your desk, or standing in a checkout line. At home, women may use vaginal weights to add muscle resistance. Talk to your clinician or a sex therapist about where to get these and how to use them.

■ **Try to relax.** Do something soothing together before having sex, such as playing a game or going out for a nice dinner. Or try relaxation techniques such as deep breathing exercises or yoga.

■ **Use a vibrator.** This device can help a woman learn about her own sexual response and allow her to show her partner what she likes.

■ **Don't give up.** If none of your efforts seem to work, don't give up hope. Your health care provider can often determine the cause of your sexual problem and may be able to identify effective treatments. He or she can also put you in touch with a sex therapist who can help you explore issues that may be standing in the way of a fulfilling sex life.

## Maintaining good health

Your sexual well-being goes hand in hand with your overall mental, physical, and emotional health. Therefore, the same healthy habits you rely on to keep your body in shape can also shape up your sex life.

■ **Exercise, exercise, exercise.** Physical activity is first and foremost among the healthy behaviors that can improve your sexual functioning. Because physical arousal depends greatly on good blood flow, aerobic exercise (which strengthens your heart and blood vessels) is crucial. And exercise offers a wealth of other health benefits, from staving off heart disease, osteoporosis, and some forms of cancer to improving your mood and helping you get a better night's sleep. Also, don't forget to include strength training.

■ **Don't smoke.** Smoking contributes to peripheral vascular disease, which affects blood flow to the penis, clitoris, and vaginal tissues. In addition, women who smoke tend to go through menopause two years earlier than their nonsmoking counterparts. If you need help quitting, try nicotine gum or patches or ask your health care provider about the drugs bupropion (Zyban) or varenicline (Chantix).

### Sex in the Internet age

The Internet is a valuable source of all types of information, including books and other products (such as sex toys) that can enhance your sex life. It has also made pornography widely and continuously available. These trends have given rise to different problems that deserve greater awareness.

The first relates to privacy concerns. Although it may be obvious, never use your workplace computer do searches for sex-related information, to avoid potential embarrassment with your employer, who is likely able to track your search history. People who feel uneasy even about using their home computers and credit cards to order sex-related information or products online might be able to find a nearby store (especially in major cities) and pay with cash.

The second is a phenomenon seen by growing numbers of sex therapists, in which people (primarily but not exclusively men) frequently view and masturbate to online pornography or participate in sex chat rooms—often at the expense of real-time sexual experiences with their partner. For some, this can become quite addictive. If you are concerned that excessive pornography use is a problem for you or for your partner, speak with your health care provider or a sex therapist.

---

■ **Use alcohol in moderation.** Some men with erectile dysfunction find that having one drink can help them relax, but heavy use of alcohol can make matters worse. Alcohol can inhibit sexual reflexes by dulling the central nervous system. Drinking large amounts over a long period can damage the liver, leading to an increase in estrogen production in men. In women, alcohol can trigger hot flashes and disrupt sleep, compounding problems already present in menopause.

■ **Eat right and maintain a healthy weight.** Overindulgence in fatty foods leads to high blood cholesterol and obesity—both major risk factors for cardiovascular disease. In addition, being overweight can promote lethargy and a poor body image. Increased libido is often an added benefit of losing those extra pounds.

■ **Use it or lose it.** When estrogen drops at menopause, the vaginal walls lose some of their elasticity. You can slow this process or even reverse it through sexual activity. If intercourse isn't an option, masturbation also is effective, although for women, this works best if you use a vibrator or dildo (an object resembling a penis) to help stretch the vagina. For men, long periods without an erection can deprive the penis of a portion of the oxygen-rich blood it needs to maintain good sexual functioning. As a result, something akin to scar tissue develops in muscle cells, which interferes with the ability of the penis to expand when blood flow is increased.

## Putting the fun back into sex

Even in the best relationship, sex can become ho-hum after a number of years. With a little bit of imagination, you can rekindle the spark.

■ **Be adventurous.** Maybe you've never had sex on the living room floor or in a secluded spot in the woods; now might be the time to try it. Or try exploring erotic books and films. Even just the feeling of naughtiness you get from renting an X-rated movie might make you feel frisky.

■ **Be sensual.** Create an environment for lovemaking that appeals to all five of your senses. Concentrate on the feel of silk against your skin, the beat of a jazz tune, the perfumed scent of flowers around the room, the soft focus of candlelight, and the taste of ripe, juicy fruit. Use this heightened sensual awareness when making love to your partner.

■ **Be playful.** Leave love notes in your partner's pocket for him or her to find later. Take a bubble bath together—the warm cozy feeling you have when you get out of the tub is a great lead-in to sex. Tickle. Laugh.

■ **Be creative.** Expand your sexual repertoire and vary your scripts. For example, if you're used to making love on Saturday night, choose Sunday morning instead. Experiment with new positions or sex toys.

■ **Be romantic.** Read poetry to each other under a tree on a hillside. Surprise each other with flowers when it isn't a special occasion. Plan a day when all you do is lie in bed, talk, and be intimate.

The most important tool you have at your disposal is your attitude about sexuality. Armed with good information and a positive outlook, you should be able to maintain a healthy sex life for many years to come. ▼

# Resources

## Organizations

**American Association of Sexuality Educators, Counselors, and Therapists**
1441 I St. NW, Suite 700
Washington, DC 20005
202-449-1099
www.aasect.org

A nonprofit professional association of sex educators, sex counselors, and sex therapists. You can get a list of therapists in your area by searching the organization's Web site.

**National Kidney and Urologic Diseases Information Clearinghouse**
3 Information Way
Bethesda, MD 20892
800-891-5390 (toll-free)
kidney.niddk.nih.gov/

This government clearinghouse provides accurate, up-to-date information about kidney and urologic diseases to patients, health care professionals, and the public.

**North American Menopause Society**
5900 Landerbrook Drive, Suite 390
Mayfield Heights, OH 44124
440-442-7550
www.menopause.org

This nonprofit organization provides general information about menopause for consumers to help them make informed health decisions. It offers a free monthly e-mail newsletter, *Menopause Flashes*, as well as an online booklet, "Sexual Health and Menopause," available at www.menopause.org/sex.aspx.

**Urology Care Foundation**
1000 Corporate Blvd.
Linthicum, MD 21090
800-828-7866 (toll-free)
www.urologyhealth.org

The Web site includes information on erectile dysfunction and a range of other adult urological conditions.

## Books

**100 Questions and Answers About Erectile Dysfunction**
Pamela Ellsworth, M.D., and Bob Stanley
(Jones & Bartlett, 2nd edition, 2008)

Written by a clinical urologist and a patient with erectile dysfunction, this book uses a question-and-answer format to describe the diagnosis and treatment of the condition. It discusses sexual health in the context of overall health.

**Enduring Desire: Your Guide to Lifelong Intimacy**
Michael E. Metz and Barry W. McCarthy
(Routledge, 2010)

This book features real-life examples and exercises designed to help couples achieve realistic sexual satisfaction.

**Sex Matters for Women: A Complete Guide to Taking Care of Your Sexual Self (Second Edition)**
Sallie Foley, Sally A. Kope, and Dennis P. Sugrue
(Guilford Press, 2012)

Written by therapists, this guide draws on current, science-based information, exercises, and advice to help women understand how their bodies work and take charge of their sexuality.

**When Sex Hurts: A Woman's Guide to Banishing Sexual Pain**
Andrew Goldstein, M.D., Caroline Pukall, Ph.D., and Irwin Goldstein, M.D.
(Da Capo Lifelong Books, 2011)

This book features information on the multiple causes and available treatments for painful intercourse in women.